MRCPsych Part 1 In a Box

Bhaskar Punukollu MBBS MRCPsych
Specialist Registrar in Psychiatry,
Charing Cross & St Mary's Higher Specialist Training Scheme, London

Michael Phelan BSc MBBS MRCPsych
Consultant Psychiatrist, West London Mental Health Trust &
Honorary Senior Lecturer, Imperial College School of Medicine, London

Anish Unadkat BMBS Bmedsci
Senior House Officer in General Adult Psychiatry,
Chelsea and Westminster Hospital, London

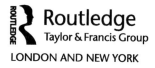

Routledge
Taylor & Francis Group

LONDON AND NEW YORK

First published 2007 by Royal Society of Medicine Press Ltd.

Published 2018 by Routledge
2 Park Square, Milton Park, Abingdon, Oxon OX14 4RN
52 Vanderbilt Avenue, New York, NY 10017

Routledge is an imprint of the Taylor & Francis Group, an informa business

British Library Cataloguing in Publication Data
A catalogue record for this book is available from the British Library

Designed and typeset by Phoenix Photosetting, Chatham, Kent

ISBN 13: 978-1-85315-602-1 (hbk)
ISBN 13: 978-1-138-11246-9 (pbk)

The aim of MRCPsych Part 1 in a Box is to help you pass your exam. The cards provide specific and up to date information, based on the syllabus and the experiences of recent candidates. They are produced for easy reading and quick learning. Mnemonics are frequently used to help you remember key facts. The box is one of the only revision aids that contains information for all components of the exam; key facts for the written and OSCEs as well as detailed practice ISQ and EMI questions.

We hope that the cards help to make your revision more effective and fun. They are designed to be taken anywhere, shared with colleagues and to bring you success!

The first nine sections of cards are broadly divided into commonly tested areas on the exam:

1. Neurotic disorders
2. Affective disorders
3. Dementia syndromes
4. Neuropsychiatry
5. Psychology
6. Psychotherapy
7. Schizophrenia
8. Pharmacology
9. Human development

Section 10 includes various miscellaneous topics which are commonly tested, including classification in psychiatry, rating scales, organic conditions and summaries of the NICE guidelines, which are useful for OSCE practice.

Section 11 covers commonly asked OSCEs. A simple 'suggested approach' is offered on how to tackle each station. Each card also includes a more in depth explanation of key areas to address on each station as well as useful tips explaining common reasons for candidates failing.

Section 12 (the last section) consists of a selection of ISQs and EMIs, exam type questions, with comprehensive answers and explanations.

2. Contents

Delusional states

- **Morbid jealousy:** delusional belief of a partner's infidelity. There is an association with alcoholism, schizophrenia, substance misuse, mania, delirium and dementia.

- **Folie à deux:** similar or identical delusional system develops in a person as a result of a close relationship with another person who has an established delusional system. The condition is rare and usually there is a dominant partner with fixed delusions who appears to induce similar delusions in a dependent or suggestible partner.

- **De Clerambault's syndrome:** a person develops a delusional belief that another person is in love with them and becomes obsessed with that person, thinking about them all the time, sometimes dressing like them and/or stalking them.

Delusions of misidentification

- **Reduplicative paramnesia:** a feeling that a familiar place has been duplicated.
- **Capgras' syndrome:** the delusional belief that a familiar person has been replaced by an imposter who looks identical or very similar to the person they know. It is more common in females and about 50% of cases are associated with schizophrenia.
- **Fregoli's syndrome:** a belief that a stranger has been replaced by a familiar person.
- **Doppleganger:** a feeling that another human being is accompanying the self.
- **Cotard's syndrome:** a delusion that one has lost some part of the body, internal organs, limbs or a belief that they are dead.

Hallucinations

- **Visual hallucination:** only seen in about 15% of people with schizophrenia. Most commonly occur in organic conditions.
- **Autoscopic hallucination:** a type of visual hallucination – seeing oneself in external space.
- **Pseudohallucination:** a percept that is experienced as similar to a real experience such as hearing a voice but it is recognized as coming from the self and is not as tangible as a real hallucination. However the person may still believe that the voice is real even though they see it as coming from inside their own head.

Hallucinations (cont.)

- **Hypnagogic/hypnapompic hallucinations:** (i) hypnagogic occur when falling asleep; (ii) hypnapompic occur when waking up from sleep. Usually these are visual or auditory perceptions such as seeing a shadow or a face or hearing a voice shouting a name. Hypnagogic hallucinations are usually brief in duration. They commonly occur in narcolepsy.

- **Extracampine hallucination:** a hallucination experienced outside the limits of the sensory field. For example, "I keep hearing someone down the road talking about me."

- **Functional hallucination:** A normal external stimulus provokes a hallucination which occurs simultaneously. For example, a patient hears voices whenever he hears cars going past on the street.

- **Reflex hallucination:** A stimulus in one sensory modality produces a hallucination in another. For example, a person sees someone walking and then hears voices. The person may then believe the person walking has led to him/her hearing voices.

Other perceptual abnormalities

- **Autoscopy:** The experience of seeing oneself and the image does not occur in external space eg they believe they see themselves in a mirror but they do not really. Schizophrenic patients may experience images of themselves in the form of a pseudohallucination. Sometimes this is called phantom mirror image. It may occur in organic conditions such as temporal lobe epilepsy or parietal lobe lesions. It is a visual perception and does not occur in other modalities. It can occur as a result of sensory deprivation. The opposite may occur – negative autoscopy – in which the patient looks in the mirror and sees no one there.

- **Lilliputian hallucinations:** visual hallucinations of small people or objects most often seen in alcohol withdrawal. These are also seen sometimes in delirium tremens.

Other perceptual abnormalities (cont.)

- **Eidetic image:** a vivid mental image is experienced in the form of a dream or fantasy. A past memory may be remembered vividly almost like a hallucination, although it is not actually a hallucination.
- **Hygric hallucinations:** the perception of fluid, eg a schizophrenic patient feels as if there is water flowing over his back.
- **Changes in the perception of shape of objects:** occur as a result of parietal lobe lesions, epilepsy, acute organic states including substance misuse (eg LSD); extremely uncommon in functional psychiatric illness although may occur rarely in acute psychosis associated with schizophrenia.

Auditory hallucinations

- **Elementary hallucinations:** This is a percept that is not specific to any part of reality, hearing non-specific sounds: eg noises, rustling or whirring. These are common in organic states such as alcoholic hallucinosis.
- Command (first person).
- Running commentary (second person).
- At least two voices speaking about the person (third person).
- Thoughts are heard out loud: (i) **echo de la pensees** (otherwise known as thought sonorization or thought echo); (ii) **Gedankenlautwerden** – own thoughts and voices occur simultaneously.

Illusions

- **Completion illusion:** Inattention leads to a misinterpretation, eg misreading a word as something similar due to inattention (eg 'word' is misread as 'world').

- **Affect illusion:** Perception of objects/surroundings/people is altered by the prevailing mood state. For example, feeling depressed about the loss of a loved one, one may see people who look similar and think it is the loved one.

- **Pareidolic illusion:** Images are seen from shapes, eg a hole in the wall is seen as shaped like someone's face. These experiences are seen in the prodromal stage of delirium tremens, or with abuses of some substances, although such experiences may also occur normally.

Delusions

Definition of a delusion

A fixed and false, unshakeable belief out of keeping with the patient's social, cultural or religious background.

Types of delusions

- **Primary:** A delusion without any possible explanation, which cannot be understood from the individual's experiences.
- **Secondary:** A delusion that arises from an understandable source such as an hallucination or a mood state, eg depression or mania leading to delusions of nihilism or grandeur.
- **Overvalued idea:** Not a delusion – an acceptable, comprehensible idea pursued by an individual but which is outside of the bounds of reason.

Delusions

Types of primary delusion

Mnemonic: I MAP

I = Delusional **I**dea (otherwise known as an autochthonous delusion) – a belief which comes from within the person and apparently arises from nowhere.

M = Delusional **M**emory – an event is remembered in a false and fixed way such that it bears no relationship to reality. Either the recalled event may have never taken place or a real event may be recalled with the sequence of events mixed up or with incorrect details.

A = Delusional **A**tmosphere/ Mood – an unpleasant feeling that something is wrong, or that something is happening.

P = Delusional **P**erception – a delusional meaning is attached to a normal percept, eg coffee tastes funny so the patient thinks this means someone put poison in it.

Symptoms associated with interruption of blood supply to the brainstem

- Cranial nerve abnormalities with or without hemiparesis and hemisensory deficits.
- Dysphagia (due to paralysis of tongue and larynx).
- Dysarthria (inability to articulate clearly due to paralysis of facial muscles).

Symptoms associated with loss of blood flow to the cerebellum

- Ataxia (motor incoordination due to cerebellar damage).
- Hypotonia.
- Dysmetria (lack of coordination of movement characterized by an inability to carry out the finger-nose test).
- Loss of equilibrium and vertigo.
- Diplopia and bilateral hemianopsia (due to loss of blood flow in the posterior cerebral artery).

Effects of anterior circulation abnormalities

Anterior circulation consists of
- Right and left internal carotid arteries.
- Pass on each side into the temporal lobe to enter the subarachnoid space. These arteries then join the circle of Willis where each bifurcates to form two main branches: **the** anterior **and the** middle cerebral arteries.
- Internal carotid arteries supply majority of the cerebral hemispheres, except occipital and medial temporal lobes, which are supplied by the posterior circulation.

Damage to the anterior cerebral artery
- Contralateral weakness.
- Sensory loss distally in the leg.

Damage to the middle cerebral artery
- Contralateral weakness.
- Sensory loss in face, neck and arm and to a lesser degree in the leg.
- If damage is in left (dominant) hemisphere, aphasia may occur.

Damage to the ophthalmic artery

- Ipsilateral monocular loss of vision.
- Homonymous hemianopsia.
- Amaurosis fugax.

Aphasias

- **Broca's:** Motor aphasia – understanding is preserved but speech is grossly impaired with pauses and inaccuracies and is laborious.
- **Wernicke's:** Sensory aphasia – loss of ability to comprehend meaning of words characterized by fluid and spontaneous speech but with incoherent and non-sensical speech.
- **Nominal:** Difficulty finding correct name for an object (also called anomia).
- **Global:** Grossly nonfluent speech as well as a severe fluent aphasia.
- **Alogia:** Inability to speak because of mental deficiency or an episode of dementia.

Temporal lobe lesions overview

● Psychiatric manifestations include a schizophrenia-like psychosis. Right medial lobe damage is associated with paranoid delusions in Alzheimer's disease.

● Dominant lobe lesions can cause deficits in intellectual functioning, communication difficulties (reading, writing, speech) and less commonly personality changes.

● Deeper lesions can cause neurological signs such as contralateral homonymous upper quandrantic field defects and a mild contralateral hemiparesis.

Temporal lobe lesions overview (cont.)

- Memory functions are represented in the hippocampal gyrus. With dominant lobe lesions, verbal memory is affected. In non-dominant lesions memory of music, faces and drawings may be affected. Pathology involving the dominant lobe may therefore present as a semantic impairment with fluent dysphasia and receptive language difficulties.

- Prosody is a non-dominant temporal lobe function. This is the meaningful intonation and stressing in language.

- Taste and smell are centrally represented in the uncus.

Temporal lobe

General functions

- Processing of auditory input.
- Visual object recognition and categorization.
- Long term storage of sensory input.

Dominant temporal lobe functions

- Perception of words.
- Process language-related sounds.
- Sequential analysis.
- Intermediate and long term memory.
- Auditory learning.
- Retrieval of words.
- Complex memories.
- Visual and auditory processing.

Temporal lobe

Dominant temporal lobe lesions cause

- Decreased verbal memory (words, lists, stories).
- Difficulty placing words or pictures into discreet categories.
- Difficulty understanding the context of words.
- Aggression, internally or externally driven.
- Dark or violent thoughts.
- Sensitivity to slights.
- Paranoia.
- Word-finding problems.
- Auditory processing problems.
- Reading difficulties.

Temporal lobe

Non-dominant temporal lobe functions

- Perception of melodies.
- Pitch/prosody.
- Social cues.
- Reading facial expression.
- Decoding vocal intonation.
- Visual learning.

Temporal lobe (cont.)

Non-dominant temporal lobe lesions cause

- Difficulty interpreting facial expressions.
- Difficulty decoding vocal intonation.
- Implicated in social skill struggles.
- Difficulty processing music (amusia).
- Decreased social cues/context.
- Poor visual imagery.
- Decreased recall of non-verbal items – shapes, faces, tunes.

Frontal lobe lesions

Have effects on

- Mood.
- Behaviour.
- Temperament.
- Abstract thinking and attention span.
- Speech.
- Motor activities.

Symptoms/signs

- Personality changes – disinhibition, apathy, poor motivation, euphoria, facetiousness.
- Poor judgement, concentration and difficulty planning tasks.
- Urinary incontinence may be a feature.
- Expressive (Broca's aphasia).
- Contralateral spastic paresis, lower than expected verbal fluency.

Frontal lobe lesions (cont.)

Symptoms/signs (cont.)

- Grasp reflex may occur.
- Mood changes have been classically described as euphoric but there may be emotional blunting.
- Primitive reflexes may reappear.
- If the lesion is near the motor cortex, or deeper projections, there may be a contralateral spastic paresis.
- A dominant lesion involving Broca's area may produce an expressive (non-fluent) dysphasia.
- The personality change may include disinhibition and overfamiliarity. It may include puns (witzelsucht) and errors of judgement.
- Other signs of frontal lobe pathology include ipsilateral optic atrophy or anosmia.
- If lesions are bilateral or in the midline urinary incontinence may occur.

Tests of frontal lobe function

- Stroop test (see card 72) – left dominant lobe lesions affect test the most.
- Verbal fluency.
- Tower of London test (see card 73).
- Wisconsin Card sort.
- Cognitive estimates.
- Six Elements test – plan and schedule six tasks in 15 minutes.
- Multiple Errands task.
- Trail Making Test (see cards 71 and 73).

Occipital lobe lesions

- May cause disturbances of visual processing.
- Complex visual hallucinations may occur with lesions involving the visual association area.
- There may be polyopia (multiple visual images). There may be visual perseveration (known as palinopia) or distortions of the visual scene (metamorphopsia).
- Lesions impinging anteriorly on the parietal or temporal lobe may cause visual disorientation with asimultagnosia (difficulty perceiving the visual scene as a unity).
- Prosopagnosia can also occur (difficulty recognizing familiar faces).

Parietal lobe lesions

Parietal lobe lesions are less likely to cause psychiatric disturbances than frontal or temporal lobe lesions.

Dominant lesions cause

1. Receptive dysphasia.
2. Limb apraxia.
3. Body image disorders (agnosias).
4. Right–left disorientation.
5. Dycalculia.
6. Finger agnosia.
7. Agraphia.

4–7 = the Gerstmann's syndrome.

Parietal lobe lesions

Non-dominant parietal lobe lesions cause

- Visuospatial difficulties with neglect of contralateral space.
- Anosognosia (ignoring paralysis).
- Hemisomatognosia (part of the body is felt to be absent).
- Prosopagnosia (inability to recognize faces) occurs if the occipital lobe is also involved.
- Constructional and dressing apraxia.

Either lobe can cause

- Topographical disorientation – inability to find one's way around in familiar surroundings.
- Difficulties in temporal awareness.
- Cortical sensory loss characterized by: astereognosis – ability to recognize objects placed in the hand when the eyes are shut; impaired graphaesthesia – difficulty recognizing numbers or letters written on the hand with closed eyes.

Tourette's syndrome

- Characterized by chronic motor and vocal tics.
- M:F = 3:1.
- Age of onset: 3-8 years of age, adult onset uncommon.
- 70% MZ twin concordance.
- **Motor tics:** Simple - blinking, grimacing, shrugging. Complex - touching, gesturing, hitting, biting.
- **Echopraxia:** - Involuntary repetition of the movements of another person may occur.
- **Vocal tics:** Simple - barking, grunting, snorting, coughing. Complex -**echolalia** (repeating other peoples phrases), **palilalia** (repeating other peoples words), **coprolalia** (using bad language in a repetitive and involuntary manner). Note that coprophagia does not occur.
- Motor tics usually precede vocal tics.
- OCD occurs in 20-60% of individuals. ADHD is also more common than in the general population.

Tourette's syndrome (cont.)

- Symptoms may be exacerbated by boredom or anxiety.
- Tics may be voluntarily suppressed for a short while until the tension becomes too great.
- Tics disappear when the patient is sleeping.
- Tics and OCD symptoms can be lifelong.
- Severity of tics in childhood does not affect severity in later life. Many cases improve despite severity of tics. Moderate to severe tics in adolescence may indicate more severe tics in adulthood also.
- Tics can be associated with streptococcal infections.
- Caudate atrophy occurs in some cases.
- Tics can occur as a result of stoke, head injury or encephalitis.
- **Treatment: Antipsychotics** – haloperidol is the most effective of available treatments. Alternatives include pimozide/risperidone/sulpiride/clonidine – reduces severity and frequency of tics. Baclofen may be beneficial in reducing overall impairment.

EEG

EEG ABNORMALITIES

- The EEG records the electrical activity of the brain. It is used mainly in psychiatry to look for the presence of an epileptic focus such as frontal or temporal lobe seizures that may produce psychiatric symptoms.
- The normal EEG consists of a number of frequencies – delta, theta, alpha and beta waves.
- Normal activity consists of theta, alpha or beta activity. Delta activity should normally only occur while asleep, if it occurs while awake it may represent a structural brain lesion.

Mnemonic – D TAB (delta waves are the slowest, beta waves are the fastest)

Delta – below 4 Hz.
Theta – 4–8 Hz.
Alpha – 8–13 Hz.
Beta – above 13 Hz.

EEG patterns associated with specific disorders

- **Epilepsy:** Absence seizures – 3–4 Hz spike and wave pattern.
- **Generalized seizures**: Bursts of spikes and waves (interictal). Fast activity during ictal period followed by generalized slowing (delta activity) postictally.
- **Schizophrenia:** Non-specific abnormalities (not diagnostic), commonly decreased alpha activity (fast wave), increased delta and theta activity (slow wave).
- **Creutzfeldt–Jacob disease:** Generalized bi- or triphasic periodic sharp wave complexes with a frequency of about 1–2 per second are characteristic in the majority of cases where the clinical picture also indicates the disorder, although the changes may not appear until late in the clinical course. These changes can occur in other conditions (eg Alzheimer's, Lewy body dementia) so are not 100% diagnostic of CJD.
- **New variant Creutzfeldt–Jacob disease:** Non-specific changes unlike in CJD.

Multiple sclerosis

- Characterized by sudden transient motor and sensory disturbances, impaired vision and diffuse neurological signs with a relapsing, remitting course.
- Usual onset in early adulthood, a little more common in females than in males.
- Depression occurs in around 50% of cases, or anxiety, elation or overt mania in about 10% of cases. Apathy is also common (not as common as depression, but more common than euphoria). Cognitive impairment occurs in about 50% of sufferers.

Multiple sclerosis (cont.)

● Symptoms may include slurred speech and incontinence, retrobulbar neuritis, cerebellar signs, eg diplopia, CNS signs including ataxia, nausea and vomiting or vertigo. Sensory deficits may occur such as quadriplegia or sexual dysfunction. Belle indifference (emotional incongruity) can occur.

● CSF may show increased gamma globulin. CT may reveal degenerative patches in the brain and spinal cord.

Huntington's Disease – see card 144.

Wilson's disease

- Rare autosomal recessive disorder of copper metabolism (chromosome 13).
- Usually presents in adolescence or early adulthood.
- Characterized by choreoathetoid movements, gait disturbance, clumsiness and rigidity.
- May manifest psychiatric symptoms including mood disturbance, delusions or hallucinations.
- Differential diagnosis: Extrapyramidal features, schizophrenia or mood disorder.
- Characterized by copper deposition in liver, brain and eyes (leading to development of Kayser Fleischer rings).

Neurosyphilis

- Characterized by malaise, skin rashes and ulcers. In later stages – skin lesions/arthritis/leukoplakia/respiratory or cardiovascular distress.
- Symptoms include tabes dorsalis, facial muscle atrophy, grandiose delusions in 30% of end stage disease cases, Argyle Robertson pupils (small, irregular and unreactive to light but react to accommodation). Tremor, myoclonic jerks, dysarthria and seizures occur in about 50% of cases.
- CSF serology/VDRL blood test (positive after 1 month but may be negative in some cases). FTA (fluorescent treponemal antibody) test highly sensitive.
- Presents with dementia in 20–40% of cases.
- Depression occurs in 20–25% of cases.
- Hypomania occurs in 10% of cases.
- May present with personality changes, psychosis or confusion/irritability.

Parkinson's disease

- Usual onset is around 60 years of age.
- Second most common neurodegenerative disease and most common cause of movement disorder.
- Basal ganglia affected with loss of neurones in nigrostriatal pathway.
- **Three main features:** (i) bradykinesia; (ii) tremor; (iii) rigidity.
- **Other features:** shuffling (festinant) gait, mask facies, tendency to fall, micrographia, positive glabellar tap test, hypersalivation, difficulty maintaining balance on turning.
- **Aetiology:** possible mutation in α synuclein gene on chromosome 4; iatrogenic causes – antipsychotic medication; Wilson's disease; encephalitis lethargica; progressive supranuclear palsy; vascular disease.

Parkinson's disease (cont.)

Psychiatric manifestations

- 50% suffer mild to moderate depression.
- Severity of disease is associated with severity of depression.
- Panic disorder and generalized anxiety disorder are common.
- Apathy is a common feature and occurs in as many as 10% of cases.
- Psychosis occurs in 40% of Parkinson's disease patients who also have dementia.
- May present with delusions (usually persecutory in nature) or visual hallucinations.
- Medication may be a cause of symptoms, eg bromocriptine, selegiline.
- Dementia occurs commonly in the late stages and affects executive function followed by visuospatial function and then memory and language are impaired.
- Pathological findings similar to those seen in the brains of Alzheimer's disease patients are sometimes seen in Parkinson's disease.

Anxiety disorders

Symptoms of anxiety

Psychological	Restlessness, irritability, poor concentration, fear of death, sensitivity to noise
Respiratory	Dyspnoea, tachypnoea, hyperventilation
Gastrointestinal	Dry mouth, epigastric discomfort, nausea, vomiting, diarrhoea
Cardiovascular	Chest pain, palpitations, flushing
Neurological	Dizziness, vertigo, numbness, tingling in extremities, headache, tinnitus, blurred vision, tremor, insomnia and nightmares
Genitourinary	Frequent micturation, erectile dysfunction, amenorrhoea, loss of libido
Musculoskeletal	Muscular aches
Psychiatric	Depressive symptoms, obsessional symptoms, depersonalization

Generalized anxiety disorder (GAD)

- Anxiety is not qualitatively different from normal anxiety.
- DSMIV and ICD 10 require 6 months of symptoms. In practice symptoms should be present on most days for at least several weeks and usually several months.
- In ICD 10 general anxiety disorder cannot be diagnosed with phobias, OCD or panic disorder. In DSMIV they may be diagnosed together.
- Important medical causes include thyrotoxicosis, phaeochromocytoma and hypoglycaemia.
- Genetic aetiology includes a higher concordance between monozygotic twins. GAD occurs in 20% of first degree relatives of patients with GAD compared to 3.5% of the relatives of controls.
- GAD occurs in anxious-avoidant personality disorder and other personality disorders.
- Buspirone and antidepressants are preferred pharmacological treatments. Benzodiazepines should not be prescribed for more than 3 weeks owing to risks of dependency.

Phobic anxiety disorders – specific phobias

Agoraphobia

- Fears occur when leaving home especially when in crowds or on public transport.
- It is more common in women and avoidance is a prominent feature.
- The age of onset is later than specific/simple phobias (childhood) and social phobia. Most cases occur in early or mid twenties. There is another smaller peak in the mid thirties. The mean age of onset is 30.
- The onset of agoraphobia is often but not always associated with panic attacks.
- In DSM IV the criteria for panic disorder cannot be met for a diagnosis of agoraphobia, ie more than four panic attacks in 4 weeks. In ICD10 agoraphobia is coded for with and without panic attacks.
- Lifetime prevalence: agoraphobia (7%) < specific phobias (11%) < social phobia (13%).
- Cognitive behavioural understanding of the formation of agoraphobia includes reinforcement of an avoidant response and sensitization to physical symptoms

General facts about specific phobias

- Most originate in childhood and anticipatory anxiety is common. The prevalence is three times greater in women. Phobias may have a modest but not a strong genetic component, eg phobia of heights.

- Locus of control theories are present for depression and not phobias. Imprinting is not a significant theory for single object phobia. Preparedness can help to explain the development of phobias.

- Psychoanalytical theories state that phobias are related to internal anxieties which have been repressed and displaced.

Social phobia

- Anxiety occurs in situations where a person could be criticized.
- Avoidance is common.
- Alcohol misuse is more common in this phobia.
- Onset usually between 17 and 30.
- Social phobia is commonly manifested in small group settings.

Other general facts about social phobia

- A behavioural assessment of phobia includes an understanding of incubation and habituation.
- Animal phobias do not occur in social phobias more than can be accounted for by chance.

Panic disorders

- Anxiety builds up quickly with a severe response with fear of a catastrophic outcome.
- There may be anticipatory anxiety.
- There must be three panic attacks within a 3-week period: (i) at times where there is no objective danger; (ii) not being confined to known or predictable situations; (iii) there should be comparative freedom from anxiety symptoms between attacks, anticipatory anxiety may occur.
- Hyperventilation can produce many symptoms.
- It is two to three times as common in women compared to men.
- Panic disorder is familial.
- Chemical agents such as sodium lactate can induce panic attacks more in people with panic disorder than in healthy people.
- Clomipramine is an effective agent in treating panic attacks. SSRIs may be used in practice because of their better side-effect profile. Benzodiazepines are sometimes required in high doses to control panic attacks.
- Peak incidence of panic disorders is in the thirties and forties.

Other general facts about panic disorders

- Rotational vertigo is not present in anxiety disorders.
- The months backwards test is normal in people with anxiety, it is a test of concentration which may be abnormal in depression.

Obsessive-compulsive disorder

- In OCD, compulsive rituals usually follow intrusive thoughts.
- Symptoms must be present on most days for at least two successive weeks, and be the source of distress or interference with activities.
- Thoughts are ego-dystonic.
- Compulsive rituals do not always relieve anxiety.
- There is a higher comorbidity with anxiety, depression and schizophrenia.
- Depersonalization may occur but not delusional beliefs.

Obsessive-compulsive disorder (cont.)

- Craving is not associated with OCD.
- The lifetime prevalence is 2–3%.
- The mean age of onset is 20.
- Studies have shown a slightly higher prevalence in women (1.2:1).
- In psychoanalytic theory, OCD may be seen as a regression to the anal stage of development.
- Clomipramine is effective, SSRIs are useful but noradrenaline deficiencies are not thought to be important in OCD.
- SSRI doses are higher than for depression and this is usually combined with CBT.
- Dynamic psychotherapy is not helpful.
- Neurosurgery is helpful in severe cases.

Eating disorders

Anorexia nervosa

- Deliberate weight loss induced or sustained by the patient.
- Body weight 15% below expected or BMI 17.5 or less.
- Fattening foods are avoided, laxatives and diuretics as well as insulin may be abused.
- Self-induced vomiting is compatible with the diagnosis.
- Endocrine disorder including amenorrhoea in women (may be masked by the oral contraceptive pill) and in men there may be a loss of sexual interest and potency.
- Seen more in monozygotic than dizygotic twins.
- Episodes of hyperphagia may occur during the illness.
- Concern about body image is not useful in distinguishing anorexia from depression.

Risk factors

- Cluster C personalities and autistic spectrum disorders are more common in anorexics.
- Life events can precipitate illness.
- It is more common in enmeshed, overinvolved families.
- Premature birth and low birth weight are risk factors.
- It is overrepresented in higher social classes I and II.

Eating disorders (cont.)

Anorexia nervosa (cont.)

Physical changes
- **Cardiovascular:** bradycardia, Hypertension, QT prolongation, arrhythmias.
- **Gastrointestinal:** swollen salivary glands, dental caries, erosions of enamel due to vomiting, delayed gastric emptying, constipation and pancreatitis.
- **Blood tests:** dehydration (raised urea), hypoglycaemia, hypercholesterolaemia, raised amylase and LFTs, reduced potassium, magnesium, calcium and phosphate. Normochromic, monocytic or iron-deficient anaemia, leucopenia.
- **Endocrine:** increased GH and cortisol, reduced oestrogen, progesterone and T_3.
- **Renal:** diabetes insipidus, renal failure.
- **Musculoskeletal:** osteoporosis.
- **Miscellaneous:** lanugo hair growth, infections, hypothermia.

Bulimia nervosa
- May have normal weight.
- Physical changes are the same as anorexia but less severe.
- Russell's sign may be present – calluses on dorsal surfaces of hands owing to induced vomiting.

Hyperphagia
- Present in both Prader-Willi and Klein-Levin syndromes.

Personality disorders (card 1 of 2)

- Result in ingrained and enduring behaviour patterns which are extreme deviations from the normal individual's behaviour in the person's culture.
- Appear in childhood or adolescence.
- Cyclothymia and schizotypal disorder are not personality disorders in the ICD10.
- Personality disorders feature on axis 2 of DSM IV.

Three clusters described in DSMIV

- **Cluster A – odd/eccentric:** paranoid, schizoid, schizotypal.
- **Cluster B – dramatic/emotional:** antisocial, borderline, histrionic, narcissistic.
- **Cluster C – anxious/avoidant:** dependent, avoidant, obsessive-compulsive.

General facts about personality disorders

- There is poor inter-rater reliability in diagnosing individual personality disorder.
- Personality disorders tend to become less prominent in later life.
- Rates of marriage and having offspring are greatly reduced.
- Prevalence in the community is approximately 3%.
- Personality disorders are most commonly found in urban males.

Personality disorders (card 2 of 2)

- **Paranoid personality disorder:** Others' actions are interpreted as being deliberately demeaning or threatening. There is an excessive sensitivity to setbacks and grudges are often held. Thoughts that conspiracies are occurring may be held.

- **Schizoid personality disorder:** There is a preference for solitary activities and there is emotional coldness. There is preoccupation with fantasies and introspection. Few activities give pleasure to the person.

- **Dissocial personality disorder:** Irresponsible and antisocial behaviour occurs. There is an unconcern for others' feelings. Relationships cannot be maintained. There is an incapacity to feel guilt.

- **Emotionally unstable personality disorder: (i) Impulsive** – There is emotional instability, a lack of impulse control and poor tolerance for criticism where violence or threatening behaviour occurs. **(ii) Borderline** – There is emotional instability, a chronic sense of emptiness, a disturbed self-image, relationship difficulties and suicidal or self-harm tendencies.

- **Histrionic personality disorder:** Excessive emotionality and attention seeking occurs. There is theatricality and a suggestible and shallow affect. Physical appearance is very important. Excitement and reassurance is sought.

- **Anankastic personality disorder:** Perfection and inflexibility are the order of the day. Decision-making is avoided. There are excessive feelings of self-doubt as well as the intrusion of unwelcome thoughts or impulses

- **Dependent personality disorder:** Others make the person's important decisions. Being alone leads to feelings of helplessness. There is unwillingness to make even reasonable demands. There is a preoccupation with fears of being abandoned by those one is dependent on.

Sleep disorders

Narcolepsy

- Disorder consists of irresistible and repeated bouts of sleep during the daytime.
- Onset aged 10–20 and rare after middle age.
- Cataplexy (loss of muscle tone) occurs in most cases but not catalepsy.
- Sleep paralysis and hypnagogic hallucinations only occur in 25% of cases.
- Family history of narcolepsy seen in one-third of patients.
- Strong emotions precipitate cataplexy but not narcolepsy.
- Schizophrenia-like disorders are more common in these patients.
- Associated with HLA DR2.
- EEG shows a rapid lead into REM sleep.
- Stimulants have an effect on narcolepsy but not on cataplexy.
- Antidepressants may reduce the frequency of cataplexy.

Sleep disorders (cont.)

Klein–Levin syndrome

- Somnolence and increased appetite can last for days or weeks.
- Long periods of normality between periods of illness.
- For further details see card 149.

Parasomnias

- **Nightmares:** This is awakening from REM sleep with detailed dream recall. Common in children aged around 5. Causes include anxiety, PTSD, fever and medications.
- **Night terrors:** Less common than nightmares and occur in children. They can continue into adult life. The child wakes up a few hours after sleeping and may be terrified and confused. Occurs in stage 3-4 of sleep. Benzodiazepines and imipramine may be used in the short term. They do not occur in PTSD or dissociative disorders as is often asked in exams.
- **Somnambulism:** There is walking or sitting up during non-REM sleep and occurs in childhood but may extend into adulthood. Sleepwalkers may injure themselves.

Post-traumatic stress disorder

- **Definition:** Delayed or protracted response to a stressful event or situation of a threatening or catastrophic nature which would cause distress in most people.
- **Symptoms:** Usually arise within 6 months of the traumatic event.
- **Features:** Hypervigilance; startle to loud noises; flashbacks and a sense of numbness; nightmares occur but not night terrors; emotional blunting may occur; poor concentration; anger; more common in women; lability of mood is not a feature.
- **Predisposing factors:** Previous history of neurotic illness or depression may lower the threshold for development of PTSD. Anankastic, dependent and antisocial personality disorders may also predispose to PTSD.
- **Treatment:** Single debriefing sessions are not thought to be useful. Eye movement desensitization (EMDS) is increasingly used. SSRIs and CBT are recommended. Tricyclic antidepressants may reduce the intrusive anxiety causing thoughts.

Adjustment disorders

- Includes psychological change to new circumstances.
- Interferes with social functioning.
- May manifest as depressed mood or anxiety.
- Rarely there are outbursts of violence.
- A child may regress to bed-wetting or thumb sucking.
- Associated with conduct disorders in adolescents.
- Onset is usually within 1 month of a stressful event.
- Symptoms do not usually last more than 6 months.
- The reaction is in proportion to the stressful situation.

Somatoform disorders

Somatization disorder

- Multiple, frequently changing physical symptoms which may have been present for years.
- More common in females usually in early adult life
- At least 2 years of multiple and variable symptoms with no adequate cause found.
- Refusal to accept advice or reassurance from doctors
- Social and family impairment due to symptoms.
- Briquets is a type of somatization disorder occurring before 30. It is more common in women.
- Patients tend to ask for treatments to remove the symptoms.
- There is excessive use of medications.

Somatoform disorders (cont.)

Hypochondriasis
- Persistent preoccupation with having a disease (not symptoms as in somatization disorder).
- Symptoms are present for at least 6 months.
- Patients demand extensive and repeated investigations.
- Patients fear medications and their side-effects.
- There is no familial predisposition to hypochondriasis.

Body dysmorphic disorder
- Patient convinced part of their body is too large, too small or misshapen. To others the body part appears normal or there is a trivial abnormality.
- Antidepressants may be of use. Surgery is usually contraindicated for the disorder.
- An increased suicide risk in this patient group.

Factitious disorder
- Patient creates symptoms to enter a sick role. This may be an unconscious process. Munchausen's is a severe form of factitious disorder.
- In Munchausen's peregrination may occur where the patient travels to another hospital presenting with the same symptoms.

Dissociative (conversion) disorders

- A disruption of the normal integration between the past, awareness of identity and immediate sensations and control of bodily movements.

- There may be primary and secondary gain. **Primary gain** is the relief gained from converting distress into physical symptoms. **Secondary gain** is when the disorder gives an advantage to the patient, usually socially, eg the patient may get time off work or not have to sit an exam

- There is usually a trigger to the disorder but this may not be identified by the patient.

- **Dissociative amnesia:** See card 140.

- **Dissociative fugue:** See card 140.

Dissociative (conversion) disorders (cont.)

- **Multiple personality disorder (Dissociative Identity Disorder in ICD 10):** There are usually two personalities or two patterns of behaviour. There are sudden alternations where the former personality is forgotten. There may rarely be more than two personalities. The patient may forget personal information and there are no organic explanations to the disorder.

- **Ganser's syndrome:** This was first described in prisoners. Approximate answers are given to tests such as simple arithmetic. There is clouding of consciousness and there may be psychogenic physical symptoms as well as hallucinations.

- **Depersonalization and derealization disorder:** Patients describe feelings of not being real. External objects may appear as if they are automated. It is an unpleasant experience which is usually associated with other psychiatric disorders but is rarely present on its own. Insight is retained and there is a change in the passage of time. It is more common in women and symptoms often appear suddenly. Depersonalization as a phenomenon can be experienced in normal people.

- Further details: see card 162.

Schizophrenia

History

- Dementia praecox coined by Morel in 1856.
- Catatonia described by Kahlbaum in 1868.
- Kraeplin distinguished dementia praecox from affective psychosis in 1896 and also further developed catatonic, hebephrenic and paranoid subtypes.
- Bleuler introduced concept of schizophrenias in 1911. The four primary symptoms which he felt were fundamental for the diagnosis are (4As): loosened **A**ssociations, **A**ffective incongruity, **A**mbivalence, **A**utism.
- Secondary symptoms were not felt to be key to the diagnosis and included hallucinations and delusions.
- Kurt Schneider stated in 1959 that in the absence of organic brain disease the first-rank symptoms were indicative of schizophrenia.

Schizophrenia (cont.)

First-rank symptoms

● Auditory hallucinations:

(i) Hearing thoughts repeated out loud
(ii) In the third person
(iii) As a running commentary
(iv) Made Affect
(vi) Made Volitions
(viii) Thought Broadcast
(x) Delusional Perception

(v) Made Will
(vii) Thought Insertion
(ix) Thought Withdrawal
(xi) Somatic Passivity.

NB There is high inter-rater reliability for first-rank symptoms.

Second-rank symptoms

● Perplexity.
● Emotional blunting.
● Other hallucinations and delusions.

Schizophrenia

Operational criteria for schizophrenia

- **ICD10:** At least one of Schneider's first-rank symptoms is required.
- **Other symptoms used to make the diagnosis, of which two are required:** Persistent hallucinations in any modality, thought blocking, thought disorder, catatonic behaviour, negative symptoms or loss of social function.
- One month of symptoms is required and these must be in clear consciousness. It must not be diagnosed in the presence of overt brain disease and epilepsy and drug intoxication must be excluded. Affective symptoms should not predominate.

Schizophrenia (cont.)

Operational criteria for schizophrenia

- **DSMIV:** Requires a total of at least 6 months in which 1 month there are active symptoms. There is a criteria-based social and occupational dysfunction during this time.
- There must be two characteristic symptoms from delusions, hallucinations, disorganized speech, disorganized catatonic behaviour or negative symptoms. Only one symptom is required if there are bizarre delusions, auditory hallucinations or voice in a running commentary.

Schizophrenia

Subtypes according to ICD10

● Diagnosis according to ICD10 is reliable (a common question!).

Paranoid schizophrenia

● This is the commonest type and hallucinations and/or delusions are prominent.
● Disturbances of affect, speech, volition and catatonic features are not prominent.
● Hallucinations occur in any modality.
● Common delusions include delusions of control, passivity and persecutory delusions.
● Primary delusions are more common in acute schizophrenia than chronic schizophrenia.
● Pareidolia is not a common feature in schizophrenia.
● Visual hallucinations are seen in only 10–20% of schizophrenic patients.

Schizophrenia (cont.)

Hebephrenic schizophrenia

- This has an earlier age of onset between 15 and 25 years.
- Affective changes are prominent and not hallucinations and delusions.
- Negative symptoms are common including flattening of affect and loss of volition.
- Delusions are often described as fleeting and fragmentary.
- The premorbid personality is often shy and solitary.
- Mannerisms and irresponsible behaviour are common.
- Catatonic features are very rare in this form of schizophrenia.

Simple schizophrenia

- There is an insidious but progressive development of oddities of conduct, inability to meet the demands of society and decline in total performance.
- Delusions and hallucinations are not evident and the disorder is less obviously psychotic than other subtypes.
- Negative symptoms develop without obvious psychotic features.
- A period of a year is required to make a diagnosis.

Schizophrenia

Catatonic schizophrenia

- Psychomotor disturbances are prominent; there may be extremes such as **hyperkinesis** and **stupor** or automatic obedience and **negativism**.
- There may be a plastic resistance to movements of the patient's body (**waxy flexibility**).
- Attitudes and postures may be maintained for a long time without much discomfort – **catalepsy**
- Catatonic schizophrenia is seen less now in developed countries than in the developing world.

Residual or chronic schizophrenia

- A chronic stage in a schizophrenic disorder where earlier positive symptoms and a previous psychotic episode meeting the criteria for schizophrenia is replaced by long term though not irreversible negative symptoms.
- There must be an absence of organic pathology and chronic depression and negative symptoms must last for a year.

Undifferentiated schizophrenia

- The conditions are met for making a diagnosis of schizophrenia but not conforming to the above subtypes.

Postschizophrenic depression

- A depressive episode occurring after schizophrenic illness.
- Some schizophrenic symptoms may be present but no longer dominate the picture.
- The schizophrenic illness should have been within the last 12 months.
- Depressive symptoms have been present for more than 2 weeks and fulfil criteria for a depressive episode.
- There is an increased suicide risk.

Schizophrenia

Epidemiology of schizophrenia

- Incidence = 15–30 per 100 000 per year.
- Prevalence is 0.5–1% (low incidence but high prevalence).
- Higher rates reported in communities in Sweden and Finland as well as Afro-Caribbean population in the UK.
- Age of onset: 15 and 45 years (approximately 5 years earlier in men).
- Prevalence equal in men and women.
- More common in social classes IV and V.
- Mortality twofold compared to general population.

Aetiology

Genetics

- Monozygotic twin concordance in schizophrenia has aetiological significance.
- The child of one schizophrenic parent has about a 13% lifetime risk of developing schizophrenia. If both parents are affected there is a 46% lifetime risk.
- Siblings of an affected individual have a 10% risk and if one parent is affected additionally the sibling has a 17% risk.
- Adoption and linkage studies have suggested likely polygenic and multifactorial inheritance with environment playing a role.

Schizophrenia (cont.)

Aetiology

Environment
- Late winter and early spring births are marginally more likely to develop schizophrenia. This may be due to increased exposure to viral infections.
- Rates are higher in urban areas.
- Families with high levels of expressed emotions can provoke relapse of schizophrenic illness in family members.
- Double bind is not of aetiological significance in schizophrenia.

Personality
- Schizotypal personality disorder is aetiologically linked to schizophrenia.

The brain in schizophrenia
- On average, the lateral ventricles are larger in people with schizophrenia. MRI has shown reduction in cortical grey matter. The frontal lobe and left temporal lobes are reduced in size. The parahippocampal gyrus is reduced in size and this is also found in postmortem studies. The hippocampus and amygdala are reduced in size particularly on the left. There may be widening of sulci and thickening of the corpus callosum.
- There is hypofontality in functional brain imaging and a decrease in blood flow in frontal and prefrontal cortex demonstrated with tests such as the Wisconsin Card Sorting Test. None of these changes are diagnostic.

Schizophrenia – aetiology

Premorbid factors

- There is a lower premorbid IQ and lower educational test scores in childhood.
- Children who go on to develop schizophrenia have delayed motor developmental milestones and have a preference for solitary play at age 4.
- Children may also show greater hostility towards adults and may have speech and reading difficulties.
- Other risk factors include a previous diagnosis of depression, anxiety, ADHD or conduct disorder.

Neurotransmitters in schizophrenia

- **Dopamine:** Hypothesis states there is excess dopaminergic activity in the mesolimbic–mesocortical pathways. All effective antipsychotics block D_2 receptors. Other evidence: amphetamines (dopamine agonists) can cause an acute psychosis; only the *cis* isomer of flupenthixol which is a dopamine antagonist has antipsychotic properties; postmortem studies reveal increased D_2 receptors in the basal ganglia and limbic system. PET studies have also suggested increased D_2 receptors in striatum.

- **Serotonin:** LSD, a hallucinogen, acts at serotonin receptors. Risperidone and clozapine are $5HT_2$ receptor antagonists. Ritanserin, a selective $5HT_2$ antagonist, reduces negative symptoms of schizophrenia when given adjunctively with antipsychotics.

- **Glutamate:** Glutamate is the major excitatory neurotransmitter in the cortex and has extensive interactions with dopamine pathways. Decreased glutamatergic function at NMDA receptors can cause psychotic symptoms as produced by NMDA receptor antagonists (PCP and ketamine).

Differential diagnoses for psychotic symptoms

- **Psychiatric:** bipolar 1 disorder, brief psychotic disorder, major depressive disorders with psychosis, schizoaffective disorder, personality disorders, adjustment disorders, delusional disorder, dissociative identity disorder, PTSD.

- **Organic:** acute intermittent porphyria, adrenoleukodystrophy, early Alzheimer's disease, congenital adrenal hyperplasia and Cushing's syndrome, epilepsy, Freidreich's ataxia, Huntington's disease, CVA, metachromic leukodystrophy, multiple sclerosis, narcolepsy, subarachnoid haemorrhage and subdural haematoma, SLE, trauma, tumours of the brain, Wilson's disease.

Differential diagnoses for psychotic symptoms (cont.)

- **Infections include:** bacterial infections, CJD, HIV, herpes simplex virus and tuberculous meningitis.

- **Nutritional deficiencies include:** folic acid deficiency, niacin deficiency, vitamin B_{12} deficiency.

- **Heavy metals poisoning:** include lead and mercury.

- **Medications:** several medications can cause hallucinations, delusions and thought disorder. However symptoms caused by medications tend to be more consistent with depression, dementia or delirium. Symptoms are usually reversed when causative medication is discontinued.

- **Illicit substance abuse:** Drugs which can produce psychosis include alcohol, amphetamines, cocaine, LSD, Ecstasy, opiates and PCP. Cannabis use tends to produce perceptual disturbances rather than true psychosis. However cannabis has a causal role in schizophrenia both in onset and precipitating the illness.

Neurophysiological changes in schizophrenia

● **EEG changes:** Include decreased alpha wave activity, increased theta wave activity, epileptiform activity with increased fast spike activity following stimulation procedure and increased paroxysmal activity.

● **Reduced amplitude of the P300 response:** This is an evoked potential which occurs 300 ms after a subject identifies a target stimulus embedded in a series of irrelevant stimuli. The P300 response is a measure of auditory information processing. Abnormalities of the P50 potential have also been noted.

● **Abnormal eye tracking in 50–80% of patients and their first-degree relatives:** May indicate dysfunction in the neural network involving the temporal areas of the extrastriate cortex. However a common exam question is whether visual scanning in children predicts future schizophrenia and this is false.

Neurophysiological changes in schizophrenia (cont.)

- **Impaired skin-conductance orienting response to novel stimuli:** About 50% of people with a schizophrenia fail to produce the response and the other 50% fail to habituate.

- **IQ:** Patients with schizophrenia may have a lower than average IQ before the illness and there is a further decline within the first few years of illness. 50% may have a normal IQ prior to development of schizophrenia.

- **Poor functioning on tests of:** Memory; language; executive functions (set shifting and forward planning). Visuospatial processing is spared. Neuropsychological impairments tend to correlate with negative symptoms.

Schizophrenia

Poor prognostic factors in schizophrenia

- Low IQ.
- Male sex.
- Single status.
- History of obstetric complications.
- Early age of onset.
- Insidious onset.
- Family history of schizophrenia.
- Negative symptoms.
- History of substance abuse.
- **General prognosis:** Approximately a third recover, a third have relapses and remissions and a third have a chronic deteriorating course.

Predictors of relapse of schizophrenia

- Stressful life events.
- High expressed emotion in the family.
- Illicit drug use – regular cannabis use is a risk factor for schizophrenia.
- Poor compliance with medications.

NB Tangentiality and formal thought disorder are not predictors of relapse.

Schizophrenia (cont.)

Schizophrenia in learning disability

- Schizophrenia is seen more in learning disability compared to the general population.
- Delusions are not usually elaborate and the patient may exhibit unpredictable and aggressive behaviour instead. Catatonic features are more common in this population.

Schizophrenia in later life

- Late-onset schizophrenia is much more common in women and occurs from age of 40 to 60. Formal thought disorder and negative symptoms are less common than the early onset group.
- Very late onset schizophrenia or 'paraphrenia' starts after age 60. It is associated with visual impairment and conductive deafness. Most common feature is persecutory delusions. Auditory, tactile and olfactory hallucinations are common but not visual hallucinations. Negative symptoms are extremely rare. The risk of schizophrenia to first-degree relatives is 3%, which is halfway between earlier onset schizophrenia and the general population.

Postschizophrenic depression

- Described under schizophrenia in ICD10.

Other psychotic disorders

Schizoaffective disorder
● Term introduced by Kasanin (1933).
● Patients equally share schizophrenic and affective features simultaneously within the same episode of illness.
● Symptoms are usually within a few days of each other. The criteria for schizophrenia or a depressive or manic episode are not met.
● A depressive type and a manic type; the depressive subtype is said to have a worse prognosis.
● Long term outcome is between that of schizophrenia and affective disorders.

Schizotypal disorder
● Classified with schizophrenia, not personality disorders, in the ICD10 (DSM IV classifies it under personality disorders).
● Not a form of schizophrenia but odd, eccentric beliefs and anomalies of thought and affect resembling schizophrenia. However schizophrenic symptoms such as hallucinations or delusions are uncommon and, if occur, are not of same quality as in schizophrenia.
● Condition may evolve into overt schizophrenia. For a full description see card 167.

Other psychotic disorders (cont.)

Delusional disorders
- Single or set of related delusions which can be persistent or lifelong.
- Often very difficult to treat.
- No schizophrenic symptoms such as delusions of control or hallucinations.
- Delusions must be present for 3 months and be should be personal rather than subcultural.
- Specific delusions (covered also in psychopathology section).

Pathological jealousy
- Person holds the belief that his/her sexual partner has been unfaithful. Person may go to great lengths including stalking and checking the partner's underwear. Couple may need to separate.
- Associated with drug and alcohol abuse, paranoid schizophrenia, depression, as well as organic brain disorders.

Erotomania
- Person holds a delusional belief that someone of a higher social status is in love with them.
- More common in women.
- Eventually rejections may turn into bitterness or animosity.
- Erotomania is not a feature of Cotard's syndrome or OCD and it is not a misidentification syndrome (these are common exam questions).

Depression

Depressive illness

- The minimum duration of symptoms is 2 weeks.
- Depression is more common in women at all age groups.
- Using DSMIV criteria it is twice as common in women.
- Depression affects the perceived passing of time.
- Mild or moderate depression can have additional somatic features; only severe depression can have psychotic features.
- In severe depression diurnal variation in mood does not occur, instead there is a pervasive low mood.
- Feelings of guilt occur in depression and this differentiates from anxiety disorders.

Depression (cont.)

Depression and sleep

- Early morning wakening helps to distinguish between anorexia and depression.
- There is reduced REM latency, ie time to reach REM stage.
- There is increased REM density during REM sleep.
- There is a reduced length of stage 4 and slow wave sleep.

Organic causes for depression

Neurological   CVA, head injury (mild depression), multiple sclerosis, Parkinson's disease, brain tumours (meningiomas), epilepsy

Metabolic   Hypercalcaemia, hypomagnesaemia, iron-deficiency anaemia, B_1, B_6, B_{12} and folate deficiencies, polycythaemia

Infectious   Hepatitis, infectious mononucleosis, syphilis, AIDS, encephalitis, CJD

Endocrine   Hypothyroidism, hyperparathyroidism, Cushing's disease, Addison's disease, hypoglycaemia, hypopituitarism

Organic causes for depression (cont.)

Neoplasms	Pancreatic cancer, carcinoid, oat cell carcinoma
Other causes	Myocardial infarction and cerebral ischaemia, SLE, rheumatoid arthritis

Drugs causing depression	
Cardiovascular	Reserpine, alpha-methyldopa, beta-blockers, diuretics, clonidine, digoxin, nifedipine
Endocrine	Corticosteroids
Neurological	L-Dopa, bromocriptine
Miscellaneous	Antimalarials (chloroquine, mefloquine), pentazocine, indometacin, sulfonamides
Substances of abuse	Alcohol
	Once withdrawn – cocaine, amphetamines, heroin and benzodiazepines

Beck's cognitive model of depression

- Beck (1976) proposed that automatic thoughts revealed **negative views about the self, the world and the future (a negative cognitive triad).**
- The automatic thoughts are fuelled by the cognitive distortions (described on card 161).
- The rules develop from 'schema' laid down in earlier life.
- See card 161 for a description of cognitive distortions as described by Beck.

Beck's cognitive model of depression (cont.)

- Sociotropic and autonomous personality traits can predispose people to depression.

- **Sociotropic personality traits:** These individuals depend upon others for approval and develop close dependent relationships. They are sensitive to rejection or loss of a relationship.

- **Autonomous personality traits:** These individuals find success in their own initiative and achievements. They react badly to setbacks which involve progress they have made, eg in their career.

Depression

Epidemiology of depression

- Average age of onset 27.
- Older people more likely to commit suicide although younger men are increasingly seen to be at risk.
- Depressed men are more likely to commit suicide than depressed women.
- It is three times higher in those divorced.
- Marriage is protective.
- Associated with the lower social class, urban areas and unemployment.

Vulnerability factors for depression

- Lack of a confiding relationship.
- Unemployment.
- Three or more children under the age of 14.
- Loss of mother before age 11.

Depression (cont.)

Genetics

- There is a 1.2- to 2-fold increase in monozygotic compared to dizygotic twins.
- There is a stronger genetic component with more severe depression.

Life events

- Life events can trigger depressive episodes.
- Humiliation and entrapment have more potential to create depression than loss.

Disruption to the normal circadian rhythm

- Sleep changes owing to shift work or long haul flights can precipitate affective disorder especially bipolar affective disorder.
- Flying from East to West predisposes more to a depressive episode, while travelling from West to East may precipitate hypomania.

Physiological changes in depression

Endocrine

Thyroid

- In a third of patients there is a reduced TSH response to TRH.
- There is an increased or normal TRH.
- There is a normal or decreased TSH.
- There may be increased thyroid autoantibodies.

Hypothalamus, pituitary, adrenal

- There is a consistently found raised cortisol secretion.
- There is an approximately 60% increase in glucocorticoid secretion.
- There is a reduced ACTH response to CRH.
- There is non-suppression of dexamethasone.

Physiological changes in depression

Monoamine theory of depression

- Three neurotransmitters have been implicated – serotonin, noradrenaline and dopamine.
- Agents that deplete monoamines can cause depression.
- Antidepressants increase serotonin and noradrenaline.
- CSF 5-HIAA is lower in patients who have had a suicide attempt.
- Plasma tryptophan (a precursor for serotonin) are lower in untreated depressed patients.
- It appears that lowering brain 5HT only produces depression in those already pre-disposed to it.
- Levels of HVA, the dopamine metabolite, are low in the CSF.
- Second messenger production and intracellular signalling may bring about the production of neurotrophins which may regulate mood.

Bipolar affective disorder

- At least two episodes of mood disturbance required in ICD10 but in DSM IV one episode of mania or hypomania is sufficient.
- **Type 1:** At least one manic episode identified. Depressive episodes usually occur but not always.
- **Type 2:** A major depressive episode is required with hypomania.

Differences between mania and hypomania

- Mania requires social and occupational dysfunction, hypomania requires less or none. In mania insight is impaired.
- Mania tends to have a longer period of mood disturbance than hypomania, mania usually persists from 2 weeks to 5 months.

Bipolar affective disorder (cont.)

- There may be prodromal symptoms which are often recognized by the patient prior to mania or hypomania. This includes sleep disturbance most commonly.
- The lifetime risk of developing BAD is 0.3–1.5%.
- Mean age of onset is 21 which is earlier than depression.
- There is an equal prevalence in men and women.
- A clear relationship to life events has not been established in mania, whereas in depression there is a six times increase in life events prior to the illness.
- Late onset bipolar disorder is rare and organic causes are important.
- The interval between episodes become shorter as the person gets older.
- The prognosis is poor for BPAD and is worse for the rapid cycling subtype.
- Bipolar type 2 has a better prognosis than type 1.
- Patients with acute mania perform badly on attention, learning, memory and executive function tasks.

Persistent mood disorders

Dysthymia

- A chronic longstanding depression of mood not fulfilling the criteria for depressive disorder.
- There may be periods where the sufferer feels well on occasions but they feel mostly low in mood.
- More common in women and those divorced.
- Most antidepressants have been shown to be effective in treatment.

Persistent mood disorders (cont.)

Cyclothymia

- Mood is persistently unstable and the disorder starts early in adult life.
- There are periods of high and low mood, not fulfilling the criteria for bipolar affective disorder or recurrent depressive disorder.
- More common in the relatives of those with bipolar affective disorder and may eventually develop into bipolar affective disorder.

Mood disorders and pregnancy

● Psychiatric illness is more common in the first and third trimesters and in those with medical problems in pregnancy.

Postnatal depression

● Risk of depression is increased fivefold after childbirth
● Different from 'baby blues' which occur for a few hours in half of females 3-4 days after delivery.
● Offspring of depressed mothers have poorer cognitive abilities.
● Risk factors include occupational instability and a lack of a confiding relationship.

Puerperal psychosis

● Much more common in patients with bipolar affective disorder or a family history of it.
● Usual onset is 2–15 days after childbirth.
● Commonly reoccurs in future pregnancies.
● Lithium or ECT are often the treatments of choice

Mood disorders and learning disability

- Those with learning disabilities may not be able to describe negative cognitions.
- Biological features of depression become more important in making a diagnosis.
- May be an increase in challenging behaviour.
- May be attempts to self-harm.
- Rate of suicide is lower than in the general population.
- May be decreased verbal output, decreased activity levels, and a changed routine of eating and sleeping.

Mood disorder in older age

- Depressive disorder is the most common psychiatric disorder in old age, however after 60 the first onset of depression is less common.

- There may be more physical or hypochondriacal symptoms as the presentation rather than complaining of low mood, as well as having a poor motivation.

- In depressed older aged patients with depressive pseudodementia there is an increased risk of later developing dementia.

Mood disorder in older age (cont.)

- Organic conditions are common causes and include CVA, Parkinson's and neoplastic disease.
- Rates of depression are increased in medical inpatients and highest in nursing homes.
- Being of an older age is not a risk factor for depression and depression in old age responds to treatment similarly to other ages.

Bereavement

- **Grief** is the psychological and emotional processes accompanying bereavement.
- **Mourning** is the cultural, social and cognitive processes that must be negotiated to return to normal functioning.
- **Bereavement** is any loss event from the loss of a relative to a cat or a house. The person is in the stage of mourning.

Normal grief reaction

- Shock, numbness or disbelief for 2 weeks.
- Irritability as well as low mood.
- Mannerisms of the dead person may be copied.
- There may be awareness of a presence of the dead person with transient hallucinations of voice of deceased.
- Somatic symptoms include sleep disturbance, tearfulness, weight loss, poor appetite and loss of libido.
- After 6 weeks symptoms improve until 6 months, there may be anniversary reactions following this.

Other mood disorders

Mixed affective disorder

● There is a rapid change within hours from depressive symptoms to those of hypomania or mania.

● As with depression, 2 weeks are required for a diagnosis.

Recurrent brief depressive disorder

● Short-lived depressive episodes (2–3 days) occur often about once a month.

● Between these episodes the mood remains normal.

● This category does not include mood disturbance related to the menstrual cycle.

Other mood disorders

Seasonal affective disorder

- Occurs in up to 10% of the population.
- Worse in higher latitudes.
- May be increased sleep and appetite.
- Two episodes are required in 2 years with no non-seasonal depressive episodes.
- There is a family history of affective disorders in half of the patients.
- Bright light treatment or phototherapy has been shown to be effective.

Abnormal grief reaction

- More than 6 months of grief, often lasting 1.5 years.
- Numbness more than 2 weeks and social withdrawal.
- Suicide attempts and more than 2 weeks off work.
- Ideas of guilt regarding the death
- Agitated depression and panic attack.
- Identification with the deceased.

Factors indicating a poor outcome and pathological grief include

- An ambivalent or dependent relationship with the deceased.
- Female gender.
- Poor social support.
- Isolation.
- Death of a child or spouse.
- Death by suicide or murder.
- Sudden traumatic death.
- Psychiatric illness, an early age of bereavement and unemployment are risk factors for psychiatric illness

Differentiating between depressive pseudodementia and dementia

Depressive pseudodementia

Partial cognitive deficits

Onset can be dated

Symptoms may develop rapidly

Low mood precedes other symptoms

Patient may not be willing to answer questions

Poor subjective memory

Problems with concentration

Disorientation suggests an organic rather than functional disorder

Very little motivation with performing tasks

MRI or CT normal

Dementia

Global cognitive deficits

Time of onset is unclear

Symptoms develop slowly

Mood may be labile

True memory problems

The patient is often unaware of their memory problems

Efforts may be made with tasks

Cerebral atrophy or ventricular enlargement occurs

Rating scales for mood disorders

Rating scales for mania depression

- **Montgomery–Asberg Depression Rating Scale:** There are ten items on a four-point scale and this measures the psychological features of depression. It is a clinician-rated scale. It is useful for detecting responses to treatment in depression.

- **Hamilton Rating Scale for Depression:** Another clinician-rated scale. It measures the severity of depression. There is an unstructured interview technique. The scale focuses on physical symptoms more than cognitive symptoms.

- **Beck Depression Inventory:** This is a self-rated inventory. There are 21 items with four to six statements for each item.

Rating scales for mania

- **Young Mania Rating Scale:** A clinician-administered scale for assessing the severity of mania. There are 11 items and it does not assess depressed mood. It is suitable for type 1 bipolar disorder.

Rating scales for anxiety

- **Hamilton Anxiety Scale:** This is used for anxiety disorders alone and is observer rated. There are 13 items rated on five scales. There are also some questions concerning depression on the scale

- **State-Trait Anxiety Inventory:** This is a self-rated inventory. The trait section describes how the patient feels during the interview and the state section describes how they feel generally.

- **The Clinical Anxiety Scale**- This is similar to the Hamilton Anxiety Scale but there are no questions about depression. It can be used for other conditions associated with anxiety apart from anxiety disorders.

Side-effects of SSRIs

Most common side-effects

- **Sexual dysfunction:** Inhibited orgasm or decreased libido. Occurs in 50–80% of patients on SSRIs and is the most common side-effect.
- **GI upset (nausea, diarrhoea, dyspepsia):** Usually resolves after a few weeks of treatment.
- **Headaches.**

Less common side-effects include

- **Anxiety:** Particularly in the first few weeks, more common with fluoxetine than other SSRIs. Usually anxiety subsides after first few weeks and there is subsequently an overall reduction in anxiety level.
- **Insomnia or excessive sleep:** SSRIs usually lead to improved sleep but some SSRIs may cause insomnia or excess sleep in some individuals. Fluoxetine is most likely to cause insomnia although uncommon. Citalopram is most likely to cause excess sleepiness although uncommon.
- **Seizures:** Rarely.
- **Extrapyramidal symptoms:** – Tremor in 5–10%. Rarely akathisia, dystonia, tremor, cogwheel rigidity, torticollis, abnormal gait and bradykinesia.
- **Anticholinergic effects:** Paroxetine may cause dry mouth, constipation and sedation dependent upon the dose given.
- **Electrolyte changes:** Rarely decreased glucose concentrations, hyponatraemia and SIADH.
- **Haematological effects:** Reversible neutropenia rarely.

Side-effects of SSRIs (cont.)

Less common side-effects include (cont.)

- Endocrine effects: Decreased prolactin level and galactorrhoea.
- Allergic reactions: Rashes occur in 4%.
- Serotonin syndrome: When SSRIs are coadministered with lithium, L-tryptophan or a MAOI, plasma serotonin levels may be raised to toxic levels. Symptoms/effects of serotonin syndrome are: diarrhoea; agitation and restlessness; hyperthermia; myoclonus; seizures; increased reflexes; seizures, cardiovascular collapse; delirium, coma, death.

SSRIs increases plasma levels of

- Some antipsychotics – haloperidol and clozapine.
- Carbamazepine.
- Ciclosporin.
- Phenytoin.
- Tricyclics.
- Some benzodiazepines.

Lithium

- **Mechanism of action:** Not fully understood. Has effects on cation transport increasing Na/K ATPase pump activity. Also increases generation and release of 5HT. It increases transmission at $5HT_{1a}$ and decreases transmission at $5HT_2$ receptors. It enhances noradrenaline synaptic uptake as well as platelet 5HT uptake. It also increases acetylcholine levels.

- **Routine investigations prior to beginning treatment:** FBC, U&Es, renal and thyroid function, ECG, weight.

- **Monitoring:** When beginning medication, start at lowest dose – 400 mg daily – and check blood lithium level after 7 days, 12 hours post dose. Therapeutic level is between 0.5 and 1.0 mmol/L. Titrate dose gradually and check level weekly until the level is within the therapeutic range. Once therapeutic range is achieved, lithium levels need to be checked every 3–6 months, renal function every 6 months and thyroid function every year.

- **Side-effects:** Polydipsia, polyuria (amiloride can be used to treat polyuria), weight gain, cardiac arrhythmias, tremor, acne, hypothyroidism or hyperthyroidism.

Lithium (cont.)

- **In toxicity:** CNS effects – muscle weakness, ataxia, tremor (coarse), drowsiness. GI upset – nausea, diarrhoea, anorexia. Disorientation and seizures, coma and death can occur if levels go above 2 mmol/L. Long term treatment may lead to nephrotoxicity. Small reduction in glomerular filtration rate is seen in 20% of patients – usually benign. Very small number of patients may develop interstitial nephritis. Lithium can also cause nephrogenic diabetes insipidus which may be irreversible after long term treatment (>15 years).

- **Contraindications:** Renal impairment, breast feeding, pregnancy.

- **Interactions with other drugs:** Antipsychotics – may increase lithium toxicity but rarely seen in practice. Diuretics – increase lithium concentration. Diltiazem/verapamil – may be rarely linked to neurotoxicity. ACE inhibitors – toxicity. NSAIDs – lead to toxicity except aspirin and sulindac. COX 2 inhibitors – toxicity. Alcohol – increases peak lithium concentration. Xanthines – increase lithium excretion. NaCl – increase lithium excretion.

Extrapyramidal side-effects of antipsychotics

● **Tardive dyskinesia:** Abnormal movements most commonly affecting the face, mouth or trunk. Lip smacking or chewing, tongue protrusion, choreiform hand movements, pelvic thrusting. Orofacial movements leading to difficulty speaking or eating food. Movements are exacerbated by stress. Tardive dyskinesia becomes more likely with longer duration of antipsychotic treatment.

● **Pseudo-parkinsonian side-effects:** For example, pill rolling tremor of hands, bradykinesia, shuffling gait.

● **Dystonia – abnormal muscle tone:** Muscles of the eyes, mouth or face go into spasm. Eyeballs rolling up in the head – oculogyric crisis can occur rarely. Abnormal head and neck movements may occur with spasmodic turning or twisting of the neck.

● **Akathisia:** A subjective feeling of inner restlessness, nervousness or agitation. May be characterized by pacing, crossing/uncrossing legs regularly or stamping feet whilst sitting down.

Other effects of antipsychotics

- **Hormonal changes:** Hyperprolactinaemia – leading to cessation of menses and galactorrhoea in women and can cause men to develop mild degree of breast swelling.
- **Weight gain:** Common, especially with olanzapine or clozapine.
- **Sypathetic side-effects:** Postural hypotension.
- **Anticholinergic effects:** Dry mouth very common.
- **Thirst:** Up to 20% of people on antipsychotics drink an excessive volume of fluids.
- Sedation.
- **Sexual side-effects:** Loss of libido, impotence.
- Skin rashes.
- **Neuroleptic malignant syndrome (rare):** Most commonly occurs with sudden increases in dose or when first starting the antipsychotic.
- **Glucose intolerance/diabetes:** Some drugs are believed to be associated with the development of impaired glucose tolerance or diabetes, eg clozapine and olanzapine.

Tricyclic antidepressants

Side-effects

- **Anticholinergic effects are most common:** Dry mouth, constipation, blurring of vision, urinary retention.
- **Cardiovascular effects:** Tachycardia, prolonged QT intervals, ST segment depression, flattened T waves, postural hypotension.
- **Neurological effects (rare):** Myoclonic twitches, tremors with desipramine and protriptyline. Paraesthesia. Ataxia. Lower seizure threshold – some tricyclics. Low risk that tricyclics would induce seizures except in people who are already at risk.
- **Allergic reactions**: Jaundice occurs rarely. Hepatitis – tricyclics can induce a fulminant acute hepatitis although this is extremely rare (0.1–1% of the population). Rashes occur in 4–5% of those treated with tricyclics.
- **Haematological effects:** Agranulocytosis, leucocytosis, leucopenia, eosinophilia are rare complications.
- **Weight gain:** Common.

NB: Tricyclics can be used to treat peripheral neuropathy.

Tricyclic antidepressants (cont.)

Drug interactions

- A serotonin syndrome can occur when tricyclics are coadministered with MAOIs. MAOIs potentiate the action of tricyclics.
- SSRIs increase tricyclic levels except citalopram.
- Alcohol.
- Antimuscarinics.
- Antipsychotics – especially pimozide and thioridazine.

Benzodiazepines

Mechanism of action

Benzodiazepines bind at sites on **GABAa receptors** leading to an increased affinity of the GABAa receptor for its neurotransmitter GABA. The increased affinity for GABA results in sustained activity of the ion channel and thus increased passage of chloride ions into neurons.

Effects on sleep

- Reduction of sleep latency (time taken to get to sleep).
- Decreased awakenings.
- Decreased time spent in stages 0 and 1.
- Prominent decrease in slow wave sleep – stages 3 and 4.
- An increase in REM latency, but a decrease in total REM sleep.
- Increase in total sleep time.

Stages of sleep

- **Non REM:** 0 = a fully alert and awake individual; 1 = early part of sleep, EEG irregular and reduced in amplitude; 2 = short regular patterns of 12-16 Hz (spindles); 3 = deep sleep, long wavelength rhythms 1-2 Hz, delta waves are common; 4 = deep sleep similar to stage 3, delta waves more common (>50%).
- **REM (rapid eye movement):** = Very deep sleep, dreams common.

Benzodiazepines (cont.)

Mnemonic for benzodiazepine effects on sleep

- **reduction in – LATS:**
  Sleep **L**atency
  Awakenings
  Time in stages 0 and 1 and **T**otal REM sleep
  Slow wave sleep stages 3 and 4

- **increase in 'Room Temperature':**
  REM Latency
  Total sleep time

Withdrawal effects

- **Commonly:** Anxiety; insomnia; restlessness, agitation; irritability; poor concentration and memory; depression; muscle aches and pains, twitches; increased muscle tension; sweating; tinnitus.

- **Less commonly:** Paranoid psychosis; convulsions; depersonalization/derealization experiences; visual hallucinations; illusions or paraesthesia.

Other mood stabilizers – mechanism of action

- **Carbamazepine:** Blocks sodium channels and potentiates potassium channels. It enhances the inhibitory action of GABA by its action on sodium and potassium channels.

- **Sodium valproate:** Interferes with calcium and sodium channels thereby enhancing the inhibitory actions of GABA and reducing the excitatory action of glutamate.

- **Lamotrigine:** Acts by inhibiting the excitatory action of glutamate.

- **Vigabatrine:** Irreversibly inhibits GABA transaminase.

- **Gabapentin:** Thought to inhibit reuptake of GABA into GABA terminals thus enhancing the inhibitory action of GABA.

Carbamazepine

Side-effects

H – Hypersensitivity – hepatitis
A – Aplastic anaemia – 1 in 20 000
T - Toxic epidermal necrolysis – 1 in 20 000

D – Drowsiness
A – Agranulocytosis – 1 in 20 000
R – Rashes
T – Transient leucopenia in about 10% of cases in first 2 months of treatment

Other side-effects – **DAN** - **D**ouble vision, **A**taxia, **N**ausea.

Drug interactions

- Antipsychotics, lithium, Ca channel blockers – may add to CNS effects.
- Decreases tricyclic and antipsychotic plasma levels.
- Affects other drug metabolism, eg phenytoin, oral contraceptive pill, as acts as an enzyme inducer.

Clozapine

Mechanism of action (receptor binding)

Clozapine has low potency at D_2 antagonism. It has a much higher potency as a D_1 antagonist and has antagonist activity at muscarinic and histamine (H_1) receptors. It has more action on D_4 receptors than most other antipsychotics.

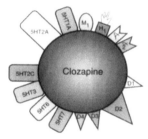

Clozapine's binding characteristics

Significant postural hypotension occurs in only 3–5% of patients on antipsychotics and is dose related. There is no reason to expect that clozapine causes less postural hypotension than other atypical antipsychotics as clozapine binds to α_1 receptors as well.

Clozapine (cont.)

Common side-effects

Mnemonic – **CASH T**o have **F**un **N**ights **W**ith

C – Constipation.
A – Agranulocytosis – risk of less than 1 in 5000 patients treated (has only ever been three deaths in total in UK from clozapine-related agranulocytosis).
S – Sedation, Seizures.
H – Hypotension/Hypertension, Hypersalivation (usually in first 4 weeks).

T – Tachycardia.

F – Fever.

N – Neutropenia – (usually in first 18 weeks). About 2–3% of patients treated with clozapine develop neutropenia. Nausea (first 6 weeks), Nocturnal enuresis.

W – Weight gain.

Psychotropic drugs – prescribing in pregnancy

Antipsychotic prescribing in pregnancy:

- A risk versus benefit analysis needs to be done when considering prescribing antipsychotics in pregnancy. Stopping the drug may lead to the mother experiencing a psychotic relapse necessitating use of higher doses of antipsychotics and increasing the risk of teratogenicity. Psychotropic drugs should be avoided if possible in the first trimester (when major organs are being formed).

- Patients who have had repeated relapses are best maintained on antipsychotics during and after pregnancy.

- The most extensively used drugs in pregnancy include: Mnemonic – **COT:**
  C – Chlorpromazine, Clozapine.
  O – Olanzapine (most widely used).
  T – Trifluoperazine.

Gestational diabetes may be a problem with both atypicals (clozapine and olanzapine). Some other drugs may be safe but there is limited data and most up to date information should be sought. It may be best not to switch to a new drug for patients who are already established on another antipsychotic.

Psychotropic drugs – prescribing in pregnancy (cont.)

Antidepressants used in pregnancy

- Again a risk versus benefit analysis needs to be undertaken. If risk of relapse is high, it may be best for patients to continue to take antidepressants during pregnancy. Tricyclics have been widely used in pregnancy without apparent detriment to the foetus.
- The most widely used drugs include: Mnemonic **– FAI** – remember the **F**ederal **A**irline **I**ndustry (FAI) of America:
  F - Fluoxetine – although some cases have been associated with early delivery and/or low birth weight.
  A – Amitriptyline
  I – Imipramine
- **Bipolar affective disorder:** Anticonvulsants are best avoided due to the risk of teratogenesis. If lithium is prescribed, a level 2 ultrasound should be performed at 6 and 18 weeks' gestation to look for Ebstein's anomaly. If valproic acid or carbamazepine are prescribed, prophylactic folic acid should be given to reduce the chance of foetal neural tube abnormalities.
- **In breast feeding – recommended drugs (Maudsley 2005 Guidelines):** Antidepressants – paroxetine or sertraline. Antipsychotics – sulpiride or olanzapine. Mood stabilizers – Avoid if possible, valproate if essential. Sedatives – lorazepam for anxiety, zolpidem for sleep.

Some other receptors associated with psychotropic drugs

Dementia drugs

- Donepezil – piperidine derivative, reversible acetylcholinesterase inhibitor.
- Memantine – non-competitive NMDA receptor antagonist.
- Rivastigmine – a butyrylcholinesterase inhibitor (reversible).
- Galantamine – tertiary alkaloid, reversible acetylcholinesterase inhibitor.

Antidepressants

- Noradrenaline Reuptake Inhibitor (NRI) – reboxetine selectively inhibits norepinephrine reuptake, with little inhibition of dopamine or serotonin reuptake. It has a low affinity for muscarinic or cholinergic receptors. It has no interaction with alpha or beta adrenergic or histaminic receptors.

- Phenylpiperizines – trazodone is a weak inhibitor of 5HT reuptake.

- Serotonin and Noradrenaline Reuptake Inhibitor (SNRI) – venlafaxine selective inhibitor of noradrenaline and 5HT reuptake.

- α_2 antagonist – mirtazapine – $5HT_2$, $5HT_3$, H_1 and α_2 antagonist. Blockade of $5HT_2$ and $5HT_3$ minimizes sexual dysfunction and nausea. H_1 antagonism effect is sedation. $5HT_3$ is a cation channel.

Psychotropic drugs

Antipsychotics

- The dopamine D_1-like receptor gene family is composed of two members, termed D_1/D_{1A} and D_5/D_{1B}:
  Risperidone – $5HT > D_2 = \alpha_1 = \alpha_2$.
  Olanzapine – $5HT_2 = H_1 = M > D_2 > \alpha_1 > D_1$.
  Quetiapine – $H_1 > \alpha_1 > 5HT_2 > \alpha_2 > D_2$.
  Amisulpiride – $D_2 = D_3$.

Classification of antipsychotics

- **Typicals:** Phenothiazines – chlorpromazine (aliphatic side chains), thioridazine (piperidine), trifluoperazine (piperazine), fluphenazine. Thioxanthenes – flupenthixol, zuclopenthixol. Butyrophenones – haloperidol, droperidol. Diphenylbutylpiperidines – pimozide. Substituted benzamides – sulpiride.

- **Atypicals:** Dibenzodiazepines – clozapine. Thienobenzodiazepine – olanzapine. Dibenzothiazepine – quetiapine. Benzisoxoles – risperidone. Imidazolidinedione – sertindole.

MAOIs

Drug interactions

- A serotonin syndrome occurs when MAOIs are coadministered with SSRIs.
- Spinal anaesthetics containing epinephrine (adrenaline).
- Antihypertensives (methyldopa, reserpine, guanethidine).
- L-DOPA.
- Narcotics – meperidine, morphine.
- Hayfever and sinus medications.
- Aspirin.
- Acetaminophen.
- Amphetamines.
- Cocaine.

MAOIs (cont.)

Foods containing tyramine that must be avoided whilst taking MAOIs

- Hard cheeses, soft cheeses. A small amount of cottage cheese is probably safe.
- Pickled or salted dried herrings.
- Hung or badly stored game, poultry or other meat which might be going off.
- Chicken liver pate and any other liver which is not fresh.
- Broad bean pods (although the beans are safe).
- Banana skins (although the banana itself is safe).
- Avocado pears.
- Food containing meat or yeast extracts.

Side-effects

- Postural hypotension.
- Dizziness, drowsiness.
- Headaches, insomnia.
- Oedema, weight gain.
- Anticholinergic effects.
- Nervousness, paraesthesia.
- Hepatotoxicity, leucopenia.
- Hypertensive crisis.

Conditioning

Classical conditioning

● A neutral stimulus is paired with an unconditioned stimulus such that the neutral stimulus causes a similar response to that originally produced by the unconditioned stimulus.

Operant conditioning

● The frequency of a behaviour is altered by the application of positive or negative consequences.

Conditioning

Example of classical conditioning

Classical Conditioning

Stage 1: Before conditioning

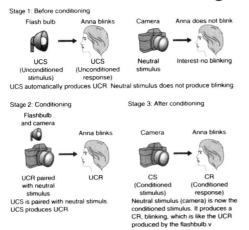

Flash bulb → Anna blinks

UCS
(Unconditioned
stimulus)

UCS
(Unconditioned
response)

Camera → Anna does not blink

Neutral
stimulus

Interest-no blinking

UCS automatically produces UCR. Neutral stimulus does not produce blinking.

Stage 2: Conditioning

Flashbulb
and camera → Anna blinks

UCR paired
with neutral
stimulus

UCR

UCS is paired with neutral stimulus.
UCS produces UCR.

Stage 3: After conditioning

Camera → Anna blinks

CS
(Conditioned
stimulus)

CR
(Conditioned
response)

Neutral stimulus (camera) is now the
conditioned stimulus. It produces a
CR, blinking, which is like the UCR
produced by the flashbulb.v

Conditioning

Example of operant conditioning

Response

Something positive occurs.

Positive reinforcement strengthens the response because it results in the occurrence of something positive.

Ellen has temper tantrum.   Alice hugs **Ellen** to soothe her.

Result: Frequency of tantrums increases

Response

Something negative removed.

Negative reinforcement strengthens the response because it results in something negative being removed or not occurring.

Ellen has temper tantrum.   Alice stops asking **Ellen** to clean room.

Result: Frequency of tantrums increases

In contrast, punishment *weakens* the strength of the response.

Response

Something negative occurs.

Punishment weakens the response because it results in the occurrence of something negative.

Ellen has temper tantrum.   Alice tells **Ellen** off.

Result: Frequency of tantrums decreases

Conditioning

Types of operant conditioning

- **Primary reward conditioning:** Most fundamental type of conditioning – learnt response is key to obtaining a biologically significant reward such as food or water.
- **Escape conditioning:** A learnt response in order to get away from a situation in which the individual prefers not to exist.
- **Avoidance conditioning:** A response to a cue is key to avoiding some type of painful consequence.
- **Secondary reward conditioning:** The learnt behaviour has no usefulness biologically but may have done previously. Eg, monkeys are taught to push a button to open a door which has bananas on the other side, the bananas are subsequently removed but the behaviour continues (ie pressing the button to open the door).

Locus of control theory

- The perceived control that an individual has over him or herself and environment.
- **Internal locus of control:** A sense of responsibility for one's own actions and a sense of being in control of own environment.
- **External locus of control:** Feeling that events are determined by external forces. Outcome (success/failure) is perceived as being independent of one's own control.
- Someone with an internal locus of control usually copes with stress better than someone with an external locus. The theory is not generally applied to specific phobias, as the cause of these is often multifactorial.

Learned helplessness – Martin Seligman

- Associated with classical conditioning.
- In Seligman's experiments, dogs were exposed to electric shocks from which they could not escape.
- The dogs eventually gave up and made no further attempts to escape new shocks given.
- The dogs then appeared to become apathetic and generally gave up on everything, not just trying to escape the shocks. The dogs displayed symptoms (apathy, helplessness) similar to those seen in human depression.
- Thus learned helplessness has been proposed as an animal model of depression in humans.
- Eg, if attempts at changing one's life are futile then the individual no longer makes any attempts to change, as they believe that nothing will help any more. This leads to a perpetuation of their depression.

Bion – basic assumptions of group work

- **Dependency:** Assuming the leader will provide all the solutions.
- **Fight–Flight:** An assumption on the part of members that there is a threat to the group.
- **Pairing:** The assumption that a new leader will arise.

Family therapy

Approach	Key concepts	Goals	Strategies used
Systemic (Milan)	Therapeutic neutrality Dirty games Counterparadox Long brief therapy	Unmasking the family game Change symptom bearers' self-sacrificing role	Therapeutic team Circular questioning Hypothesizing Invariant prescriptions Counterparadoxical interventions Prescribed rituals
Structural (Minuchin)	Boundaries Hierarchies Coalitions and alliances Complementarity Engagement–enmeshment	Increased flexibility Adaptability to developmental change. Balance between connectedness and differentiation Subsystem functioning	Multidirected Family of origin sessions Use of cotherapy
Strategic (Haley)	Power and control Family life cycle Symptom-maintaining sequences Function of problems	Resolve presenting problem Disruption of problem-maintaining sequences	Persuasion Paradoxical injunction Insight downplayed Pretend and ordeal techniques

Learning theory – definitions

- **Aversive conditioning:** Punishment or an aversive stimulation is used to reduce the frequency of a target behaviour.
- **Avoidance learning:** A form of operant conditioning in which an individual learns to avoid certain responses which result in an unpleasant effect.

Reinforcement schedules associated with operant conditioning

- **Continuous reinforcement:** A reward is given every time a response is given.
- **Partial reinforcement:** Responses are not given every time a desired response is made, hence extinction may occur (see card 70 for explanation of extinction).
- **Variable ratio reinforcement:** A reward is given after variable numbers of responses have been given – the most powerful reinforcement technique and used in casinos (eg the person playing on a slot machine may initially receive a win after five attempts, then tries again and receives a win after 16 tries, then after 11 tries, ie variable).
- **Fixed interval reinforcement:** A reward is given after fixed time periods, eg every 10 minutes.
- **Variable interval reinforcement:** A reward is given after variable time periods, eg the person on a slot machine receives rewards after 10 minutes, 16 minutes, 8 minutes, 22 minutes (so completely variable).

Learning theory – definitions

- **Higher order conditioning:** Associated with classical conditioning – a newly introduced conditioned stimulus is associated with an established unconditioned stimulus so that it produces the same response (conditioned response).
- **Habituation:** A response to a stimulus reduces with time.
- **Modelling:** Learning by observation of other's behaviour.
- **Shaping:** Reinforcing increasingly accurate responses to a desirable behaviour. Eg, In training a monkey to press a button which opens a door, initially the monkey approaching the button is rewarded. Then when the monkey touches the button, further rewards are given until the monkey finally learns to press the button.
- **Chaining:** Similar to shaping but involves reinforcing a number of simple behaviours separately and then linking them together in a more complex series.
- **Extinction:** A learned response gradually decreases in frequency once the reinforcer is removed.

Learning theory – definitions

- **Law of effect:** The principle that behaviours associated with pleasant results are strengthened whereas behaviours associated with unpleasant results are weakened.

- **Covert sensitization:** Reducing the frequency of a behaviour by associating it with imagination of unpleasant consequences – eg this technique can be used in treating sex offenders by associating an unpleasant thought with urges that the individual has to commit a sexual assault.

- **Primary reinforcer:** A stimulus that is considered to be inherently reinforcing and affects a biological process, eg affection, food, sleep.

- **Secondary reinforcer:** Stimuli that reinforce behaviour through association with a primary reinforcer.

Psychometric tests

Comprehensive trail making test

- Reliable and valid new psychometric instrument.
- Operationally defines important components of executive function.
- Consists of a standardized set of five visual search and sequencing tasks influenced by attention, concentration, resistance to distraction and cognitive flexibility (or set-shifting).

Comprehensive trail making test (cont.)

- Main uses include evaluation and diagnosis of brain injury and other forms of central nervous system dysfunction.
- More specific purposes include the detection of frontal lobe deficits; problems with psychomotor speed, visual search and sequencing, and attention; and impairments in set shifting. The basic task of trail-making is to connect a series of stimuli (numbers, expressed as numerals or in word form, and letters) in a specified order as fast as possible. The score derived for each trail is the number of seconds required to complete the task.
- The test is highly sensitive to neurological disease, injury or dysfunction, including the subtle neuropsychological dysfunction often present in individuals with learning disabilities.

Psychometric tests

- **Halstead Reitan Neuropsychological Battery:** A set of tests that examines language, attention, motor speed, abstract thinking, memory and spatial reasoning and can be used to produce an overall assessment of brain function.

- **Luria Nebraska Neuropsychological Battery:** A set of several tests designed to cover a broad range of functional domains and to provide pattern analyses of strengths and weaknesses across different areas of brain function.

- **Minnesota Multiphasic Personality Inventory (MMPI-2):** Personality assessment often used to accompany neuropsychological tests to assess personality and emotional status that might help in understanding individual's reactions to neurofunctional impairment.

Psychometric tests (cont.)

- **North American Reading Test (NART):** Reading test used to help assess premorbid intelligence, for comparison with current intelligence as measured by more comprehensive tests.
- **Ray Osterrieth Complex Figure Test:** Analyses areas of visuospatial ability and memory in all ages.
- **Rivermead Behavioural Memory Test:** Evaluates impairments in memory related to everyday real life situations.
- **Rorschach Test:** Inkblot test used to evaluate complex psychological dynamics. Useful as a complementary assessment aid in brain injury victims.
- **Stroop Test:** Brief procedure examining mental speed and control.

Psychometric tests

- **Bender Visual Motor Gestalt Test:** Evaluates visual-perceptual and visual-motor functioning, revealing possible signs of brain dysfunction, emotional problems and developmental maturity.

- **Thematic Apperception Test:** Projective test most widely used to examine personality characteristics that may aid in understanding psychological or emotional adjustment to brain injury.

- **Tower of London:** For all ages, assesses higher-level problem solving, valuable for examining executive functions and strategy planning.

Psychometric tests (cont.)

- **Trail Making Tests:** These tests measure attention, visual searching, mental processing speed, and the ability to mentally control simultaneous stimulus patterns. These tests are sensitive to global brain status but are not so sensitive to minor brain injuries. See card 71 for details of the Comprehensive Trail Making Test.

- **Wisconsin Card Sorting Test:** Measures the ability of an individual to learn concepts. It is a good measure of the integrity of frontal lobe functioning.

- **Continuous Performance Test:** Test requiring intense attention to a given visual-motor task. Used in assessing sustained attention and freedom from distractibility.

Cognitive dissonance

- Incongruity or inconsistency between two separately held thoughts, beliefs or views which are held at the same time. The assumption is that this situation cannot continue to exist, due to the distress this causes the individual. The beliefs/views are therefore reviewed and reappraised in such a way that the dissonance is lessened.

- Reappraisal may consist of changing one's notions of the opposing views by either deciding to accept one of the views and ignoring the other or searching for support from others about one of the views so achieving 'consistency'. Alternatively consistency may be achieved by changing behaviour to suit one of the views.

Emotion

- **Cannon-Bard Theory:** Cortical perception is thought to affect emotion and this then leads to secondary physiological changes which in turn further affect emotions. The emotion and physiological effects may occur quite separately and at different times.

- **James-Lange Theory:** The individual's perception of physiological changes leads to specific emotional responses. However this theory has been contested on the basis that people can react differently to the same perceived physiological changes and that sometimes emotions come before physiological changes.

Gestalt principles – perceptual organization

- Objects and figures in our surroundings are interpreted by the brain by making a number of groupings and predicting the whole figure based on the fragments. Irrelevant information from the field of vision is discarded so that the brain is not inundated with useless information. Errors in this process may lead to illusions or hallucinations.

- General principles:
  The whole is greater than the sum of its parts.
  Law of continuity – interrupted lines are seen as flowing in a continuous way.
  Law of proximity – items directly next to each other are perceived as being together.
  Law of similarity – similar items are grouped together.
  Law of closure – gaps are filled in when viewing an incomplete object so that it appears as a whole

- Figure ground differentiation is an innate skill which allows objects to be differentiated from the background and can occur in any sensory modality.

Defence mechanisms

Mature

- **Altruism:** Doing good to others (and not at the expense of one's own happiness).
- **Humour:** Expressing feelings that are difficult to bear in such a way as to avoid distress to self or to others.
- **Sublimation:** Instincts are channelled rather than dammed up inside. For example, aggression is directed into sports and games.
- **Suppression:** A conscious or semiconscious decision to postpone attention to a conscious impulse or desire.

Immature/primitive

- **Idealization:** Unconscious ambivalent desires are split into good and bad representations.
- **Introjection:** The qualities of an object are internalized.
- **Splitting:** (Klein described splitting and projection as defence mechanisms occurring in the paranoid schizoid position.) Objects are divided into all good or all bad, idealized or denigrated.
- **Projective identification:** The person projects a denied part of him/herself not so much on to but 'into' another person and ends up by powerfully controlling the receiver from within like a glove puppet (Cynthia Rogers, 1987). The denied part can be good or bad.
- **Passive aggression:** Expressing aggression towards others through passivity, masochism or turning against the self.
- **Turning against the self:** Unacceptable aggression towards others is directed towards the self.
- **Autistic fantasy:** Engaging in self-retreat in order to resolve conflict or to obtain gratification. Interpersonal communication and intimacy are restricted.
- **Acting out:** Expressing an unconscious desire through actions. Acting out is a way of dealing with an unconscious thought that is associated with an unpleasant accompanying affect.

Neurotic defence mechanisms

- **Denial:** Avoiding a painful aspect of reality by attempting to abolish it from existence.
- **Dissociation:** Temporarily but significantly changing a person's character in order to avoid emotional distress. Seen in dissociative fugue/conversion disorders.
- **Displacement:** Shifting an emotion or drive from one idea on to another which is similar to the original.
- **Intellectualization:** Using intellectual thoughts or ideas excessively to avoid distressing emotional experiences. The person may avoid intimacy by placing excess importance on inanimate intellectual items. Attention is given excessively to external reality in order to avoid expression of inner feelings.
- **Isolation:** Splitting off an idea from the unpleasant feeling(s) that accompany it (repressed feelings).
- **Reaction formation:** Behaving in a way that is opposite to unacceptable instinctual impulses.

Neurotic defence mechanisms

- **Rationalization:** Rational explanations are offered for unacceptable behaviour in an attempt to avoid the unpleasant feelings associated with facing the reality that the behaviour was wrong.

- **Regression:** Abandoning adult functioning and going back to a child-like state. This can be healthy sometimes but not when it is excessive and in the context of everyday life. Adults may regress to a child-like state following the death of a loved one for example.

- **Repression:** Unpleasant feelings are removed or prevented from entering consciousness.

- **Somatization:** Unpleasant unconscious feelings are manifest in the form of physical complaints.

- **Undoing:** Most common in people with OCD. Often referred to as 'magical undoing'. The person has unpleasant thoughts that he/she feels they have perpetrated and will then say or do something in order to reverse this wrongdoing.

- **Identification with the aggressor:** In order to deal with the pain of being treated badly by someone, the person treats someone else similarly badly. Such a mechanism is thought to occur in parents who themselves were abused in their childhood and subsequently go on to abuse their own children.

Defence mechanisms in specific conditions

Obsessive-compulsive disorder – mnemonic: U R I

Magical Undoing.
Reaction formation.
Isolation.

Paranoid states and borderline personality disorder – mnemonic: P S

Projective identification.
Splitting.

Phobic disorders

● Affective displacement.

Anxiety disorders –mnemonic: D I P

Denial.
Identification.
Projection.

Freud's models of the mind

Structural model

- **Id:** Instinctual drives – hunger, sex, aggression.
- **Ego:** The part of the mind involved in rational thinking and acts as a go-between serving to balance the demands of the Id against the superego and the expectations of the outside world.
- **Superego:** Part of the mind which carries moral values and is related to ingrained parental figures.

Topographical model

- **Conscious:** Part of the mind in which perceptions coming from the outside world are brought into awareness.
- **Preconscious:** Mental events and processes brought into the mind by focusing attention. Secondary process thinking occurs in the preconscious and conscious (utilizes logic).
- **Unconscious:** Closely related to instinctual drives. Dynamic system operating to keep mental contents and processes from conscious awareness through censorship or repression. Primary process thinking occurs in the unconscious (as in dreams).

Melanie Klein

- Studied her own childrens' play. The childrens' play activity was interpreted from an early age (1-2 years) as having symbolic meaning in the context of the unconscious mind. Klein was the first psychoanalyst to view children's play as a meaningful activity. Klein viewed infantile 'phantasy' as an important part of development. She also developed the concept of projective identification in her theories and described the 'death instinct' which she related to instinctual drives.

- Klein describes the earliest stages of infantile psychic life in terms of successful completion of development through **two positions – paranoid-schizoid** and **depressive positions**. A position is a set of psychic functions that correspond to a phase of development, appearing during the first year of life and which can be reactivated at any time later on in life.

Melanie Klein (cont.)

- **Paranoid-schizoid position:** Objects are divided into all good or all bad in the process of 'splitting' (an unconscious process). Splitting occurs in the ego and in the object. Objects are 'part objects' such as the mother's breasts which may be split into the 'good breast' which provides the milk and the 'bad breast' which does not provide milk. The paranoid-schizoid position is named as such because Klein postulated that infants in this position are in a constant state of paranoid anxiety.

- **Depressive position:** Klein postulated that the infant moved into the depressive position by about 6 months of age. The infant learns unconsciously to recognize that good and bad can coexist and no longer splits all objects into either all good or all bad. Klein describes a depressive anxiety that the infant has about his/her own aggressive feelings towards the caregiver during this ambivalent period. The mother is no longer split into internal and external objects and this creates the state of depressive anxiety (not the same as depression/anxiety in adulthood).

- Klein described that a person remains in a state of flux between the paranoid-schizoid position and the depressive position throughout their life. People in paranoid states such as psychosis or extreme anxiety may revert to the paranoid-schizoid position utilizing primitive defence mechanisms of splitting and projective identification.

C.G. Jung – Theory of Mind

- **Collective unconscious:** Expanded on Freud's concept of the unconscious, describing a topographical model with a 'collective unconscious' consisting of all humankind's common shared mythological and symbolic past. Jung rejected Freud's concepts about infantile sexuality and rejected the structural model.

- **Archetypes:** The collective unconscious contains archetypes – images that represent these mythological and symbolic aspects of humans past. Such archetypes include the image of the mother, father, hero, shadow and several others.

- **Complexes:** Archetypes are associated with 'complexes' – ideas that result from personal experiences and affected by archetypes. For example, a child may have an archetypal unconscious image of what a father is. His actual experience of his father and how it relates to the archetypal image affect the formation of a 'complex' in the child's mind. Jung was not involved in developing concepts such as inferiority complex (a common exam question).

C.G.Jung – theory of mind (cont.)

- **Personality types:** Jung noticed two types of personality – introversion and extroversion. Introverts focus on their inner world of thoughts and emotions, Extroverts focus on the outer world, other people and material items.

- **Persona:** Jung described the persona – a mask covering the personality – the face the person presents to the outside world. The persona may become fixed and the real person can become hidden from the person.

- **Animus and Anima:** Unconscious traits held by women and men respectively and that contrast with the persona. Animus – woman's undeveloped masculinity, Anima – man's undeveloped femininity.

- **Individuation –** the aim of Jungian therapy is for people to accomplish their full creative potential. This state is referred to as individuation – the process by which a person attains a unique sense of their identity.

Cognitive behavioural therapy in depression

- 16–20 sessions.
- **Initial Aim:** Assessment and problem identification.

Techniques: Behavioural

- Behavioural assignments are given to tackle motivational and behavioural deficits.
- Activity scheduling – a plan looking at relationship between activity and mood.
- Mastery and pleasure tasks – self-monitoring of degree of pleasure/sense of mastery associated with activity – an antidote to dichotomous thinking.
- Graded task assignments – breaking goals into subtasks.
- Relapse prevention work.

Techniques (cont.)

Cognitive

- Identifying and modifying negative automatic thoughts – evidence looked at/alternative explanations offered/advantages and disadvantages to a way of thinking/errors in thinking, eg dichotomous thinking.
- Identifying and modifying dysfunctional beliefs – How did I develop these beliefs? In what ways are these beliefs unhelpful?
- Guided discovery – Patient discovers problems for themselves.
- Socratic questioning – Designed to promote insight and rational decision-making.

Factors associated with a successful outcome from CBT

- Acceptance of the cognitive model.
- Willingness to engage in self-help assignments.
- Ability to form a collaborative alliance with the therapist.

Cognitive analytic therapy

- 16–24 sessions.
- Based on 'reciprocal role repertoires' – templates stored early on, eg victim/bully, abandoning/abandoned.
- People with borderline personality disorder tend to switch rapidly between roles due to a compromised capacity for self-reflection.
- The therapist focuses on recurrent faulty sequences which arise from reciprocal roles and points out the symptomatic consequences of these.

Brief psychodynamic psychotherapy

- 10–25 sessions.
- Aims to bring unconscious emotions and motivations into the conscious mind.
- Effectiveness is enhanced by:
    —An early positive therapeutic alliance.
    —Extent of therapist activity.
    —Prompt addressing of negative transferences.
    —Focused work with intrapsychic and interpersonal conflict of central importance to patients.

Cognitive behavioural therapy in psychosis

Main aims are

1. **Engagement:**
   —Obtain a therapeutic alliance.
   —Be non-challenging.
   —Listening.
   —Offer practical coping strategies for distressing symptoms such as auditory hallucinations or delusions.

2. **Gain a sense of the person's experience of their illness:**
   —Onset and duration of symptoms such as voices.
   —Explore beliefs formed from jumping to conclusions.

3. **Discover if there is a delusional mood state:**
   —Externalizing bias.
   —Delusions of reference.

Main aims are (cont.)

4. Reduce stress level through psychoeducation:
—Modifying beliefs.
—Offer alternative explanations and suggest coping strategies along with these.

5. Check patient has accepted that the brain can make mistakes:
—Once patient has accepted this concept, it may be possible to begin to modify their beliefs.

Lewy body dementia

- M>F. Onset usually in sixties or seventies.

- Presents initially with extrapyramidal features, dementia or psychotic symptoms. As disease progresses, dementia and extrapyramidal features increase.

- Dementia is mainly of cortical type with progressive worsening of memory and development of dysphasia, dyscalculia and dyspraxia.

- Day-to-day fluctuations in mental competence are observed in many sufferers. Lucid periods with near normal memory are seen until late in the course of the disease.

- Prominent behavioural disturbances with psychotic symptoms, including auditory and visual hallucinations, are common.

- Paranoid delusions and severe depression may also occur.

Lewy body dementia (cont.)

- Parkinsonian features are common – rigidity, tremor and bradykinesia, mask-like facies and stooped posture.
- Postural hypotension and falls as well as unexplained loss of consciousness are frequently seen.
- Acute organic reactions are seen including acute confusional states.
- Fluctuating course as well as visual/auditory hallucinations and clouding of consciousness distinguish Lewy body dementia from Alzheimer's disease. Depression is also more common than in Alzheimer's. Patients with Lewy body dementia do worse on tests of frontal lobe function and visuospatial tasks compared to Alzheimer's disease sufferers.
- Lewy body patients are highly susceptible to reactions from neuroleptics such as haloperidol or chlorpromazine, which should therefore be avoided.
- **Pathological findings:** Lewy bodies (rounded eosinophilic inclusions within neurones) in the cortex, substantia nigra, brainstem nuclei and basal forebrain regions.

Multi-infarct dementia

- M=F.
- Usual onset – late sixties or seventies.
- There is usually a history of hypertension, stroke or MI or other vascular disease. Onset is usually sudden and following on from a vascular event.
- If onset is gradual, personality changes often precede onset of memory changes.
- Physical complaints are common including headaches, dizziness, tinnitus or syncope.
- Clouding of consciousness as well as fluctuations in severity of cognitive impairments are common features.

Multi-infarct dementia (cont.)

- Personality may be well preserved until late in the disease. Patchy psychological deficits are common however.
- Most important characteristic – stepwise progression of illness, unlike in Alzheimer's disease where there is a smoother progression of the illness.
- **EEG changes:** Similar to Alzheimer's disease. Early in disease, reduction of alpha activity occurs. Later in the disease, diffuse slow waves occur, usually irregular theta activity with episodic delta activity.
- **Pathology:** Localized or generalized atrophy, ventricles may be dilated. Both small and large vessels are affected with thickened walls and tortuous appearances. Arteriosclerotic changes are likely to be seen in the body.
- Difficult to distinguish between multi-infarct dementia and Alzheimer's disease. Multi-infarct dementia is more likely if there is a fluctuating course, stepwise deterioration, history of ischaemic vascular event/disease, associated neurological symptoms/signs. The Hachinski Ischaemic Index can be used to distinguish between them.

Pick's disease

- F>M. Relatively uncommon (around 1-5% of all dementias).
- Peak onset 50–60 years of age (earlier than Alzheimer's disease).
- Initial features include changes suggestive of frontal lobe damage, with changes in personality and social behaviour.
- Amotivation and changes in behaviour with socially inappropriate or insensitive behaviour. Social misconduct and poor judgement leading to stealing or sexual misadventures may occur.
- As the disease progresses, memory and intellectual impairment become prominent.
- Mood changes including fatuous affect, euphoria or apathy may be interspersed between periods of restlessness and overactivity.

Pick's disease

- Perseveration of speech with stereotyped repetition of short words or phrases is common.
- Dyphasia may occur and can progress to incoherent words or mutism.
- Certain features distinguish Pick's disease from Alzheimer's – see card 163.
- EEG: May be normal and less often shows abnormalities compared to Alzheimer's disease. Non-specific changes usually occur which may be similar to the picture in Alzheimer's disease.
- Pathology: Pick bodies – irregular filamentous inclusions within neurones, which are argentophilic and immunoreactive to tau and ubiquitin antibodies occur. Hirano bodies – eosinophilic inclusions may occur. Ventricular dilatation, generalized atrophy and shrinking of temporal and frontal lobes may occur.

Frontal lobe dementia

- M=F. Usual onset in fifties.
- Characterized by personality changes with disinhibition, impulsivity, poor judgement, inability to carry out tasks and apathy. They may be socially inappropriate with lack of empathy for others.
- Perseveration and utilization behaviour (tendency to pick up anything within the visual field to play with).
- Tendency for excess oral satisfaction – overeating, eating sweets excessively.
- About 35% have a family history. Otherwise aetiology unclear. Possible association with chromosome 17 has been suggested.
- **Pathology:** Frontal lobe atrophy, cellular loss in layers III and IV of the cortex.

Creutzfeld–Jakob disease (CJD)

- Characterized by memory changes, confusion and disorientation initially. As the disease advances, a slowly worsening dementia develops. Cerebellar ataxia and choreoathetoid movements may occur. Myoclonus occurs in around 80% of cases. Extrapyramidal signs, dysarthria, akinetic mutism and cortical blindness may develop.

- M=F. Usual age of onset is over 40. Extremely rare – only 1-2/million population.

- 90% of cases are due to spontaneous mutations in the prion protein on chromosome 20 – these are referred to as sporadic CJD. Prion is a protein particle that is infectious and very resistant to degradation. Cognitive changes occur earlier in sporadic CJD compared to new variant CJD (nvCJD). Sporadic CJD also tends to affect younger people more often than nvCJD. Other types include familial (incomplete penetrance means carriers prognosis is better than in sporadic CJD and will likely live much longer) and iatrogenic (corneal graft procedures). nvCJD usually lasts longer (10–15 months) than CJD (4-5 months).

- New variant CJD occurs in a younger age group (around age 30) and is associated with consumption of beef infected with bovine spongiform encephalopathy (BSE, popularly termed 'mad cow disease' by the press). It is usually characterized by a prodrome of depression (most common), anxiety, apathy or aggression. Only about 15% have neurological problems, unlike in sporadic CJD where these symptoms are much more common. Eventually cerebellar ataxia, myoclonus and dementia develop.

Alzheimer's dementia

- Most common dementia representing about two-thirds of all dementias.

- Characterized by mnemonic **5 A's** – **A**mnesia (memory loss), **A**phasia (or dysphasia), **A**praxia (or dyspraxia), **A**nomia, **A**pathy commonly. Frontal lobe involvement may lead to symptoms mentioned on card 86. Apathy occurs early on in the illness while insight is relatively well preserved. As the disease progresses, apathy and behavioural and psychological symptoms of dementia become more common. Psychosis occurs in 20–25% of cases in the first year from diagnosis and 50% in the first 4 years.

- Prevalence is approximately 0.5% in 60–70 year olds and 10% in 80–90 year olds. Average life expectancy is 5–10 years. Poor prognosis is associated with early onset, severe cognitive dysfunction and psychiatric symptoms including psychosis or depression.

- **Risk factors include:** Increasing age, family history of Alzheimer's disease or Parkinson's disease, mild cognitive impairment, head injury, learning disability, Down's syndrome, vascular disease or risk factors for vascular disease.

Alzheimer's dementia (cont.)

- **Protective factors include:** High educational attainment, smoking, non-steroidal anti-inflammatory drugs (NSAIDs).

- **Pathological findings:** Neurofibrillary tangles containing tau protein and amyloid plaques containing amyloid. Neurofibrillary tangles are not specific for Alzheimer's and occur in subactue sclerosing panencephalitis as well as dementia pugilistica (punch drunk syndrome). Amyloid plaques also occur in normal ageing, CJD and Down's syndrome. Lewy bodies, Hirano bodies, granulovacuolar degeneration of neurones and astrocyte proliferation also occur.

- **Genetic factors:** Apoliprotein E4 (on chromosome 19) is associated with a 20 times greater chance of developing the disease if homozygous or 5% increased chance if heterozygous. Age of onset decreases with increasing numbers of Apo E4 alleles. Mutation in amyloid precursor gene on chromosome 21 is associated with early onset familial Alzheimer's disease in 20% of cases. May be inherited in an autosomal dominant fashion. Presenilin gene 1 on chromosome 14 and presenilin gene 2 on chromosome 1 have also been implicated in early onset Alzheimer's disease.

Erickson's stages of social and psychological development

Age	Stage
Infancy	Trust vs. mistrust
2–3	Autonomy vs. shame and doubt
3–5	Initiative vs. guilt
6–11	Industry vs. inferiority
Adolescence	Identity vs role confusion
Early adulthood	Intimacy vs. isolation
Middle age	Generativity vs. stagnation
Old age	Integrity vs. Despair

Freud's stages of human development

Age	Stage	Features
Birth to 1 year	Oral phase	Gratification via oral means
1–3	Anal phase	Gratification via defecation
3–5	Phallic phase	Expansion of oedipal fantasies
5–12	Latent phase	Infantile stage of sexuality ends with repression of Oedipus complex
12–20	Puberty	Sexual drives are reawoken

Freud believed that in order to function normally as an adult, it is necessary for an individual to pass through each of these stages successfully.

Developmental milestones

Birth to 1 month:

- Hand to mouth reflex.
- Grasping reflex.
- Rooting reflex.
- Moro reflex.
- Babinski reflex.
- Responds to mother's face.

4 months

- Holds head balanced without aid from others.
- Visual accommodation.
- Follows a moving object.
- Aware of strange situations.
- Spontaneous social smile.

7 months

- Sits steadily.
- Stranger anxiety begins and is established by 8 months.
- Grasps and transfers toys.
- Starts to imitate mother's sounds and actions.

1 year

- Walks with support.
- Starts to use single words.
- Stands alone briefly.
- Seeks novelty.

Developmental milestones (cont.)

18 months
- Coordinated walking.
- Walks up stairs with one hand held.
- Builds a tower of three or four cubes.
- Scribbles spontaneously and imitates writing.
- Builds tower of three cubes.
- Two-word utterances.
- Understands 150 words.

2 years
- Runs without falling.
- Kicks large ball.
- Goes up and down stairs alone.
- Builds a tower of six/seven cubes.
- Able to use sentences.

- Separation anxiety starts to go away.
- Refers to self by name and says 'no' to mother.

3 years
- Rides tricycle.
- Puts on shoes and able to undo buttons.
- Alternates feet going up steps.
- Feeds self unassisted.
- Builds tower of 9–10 cubes.
- Understands up to 3500 words.

4 years
- Able to stand on one foot.
- Repeats four digits.
- Understands wide range of grammar.

- Counts three objects.
- Copies a cross.

5 years
- Skips using feet alternately.
- Dresses and undresses unassisted.
- Able to tell a story.
- Counts ten objects correctly.
- Copies a square.
- Draws a recognizable person.
- Writes few letters.

6 years
- Rides two-wheel bicycle.
- Ties shoelaces.
- Good articulation of ideas/thoughts.
- Copies triangle.
- Writes name.

Margaret Mahler – separation individuation stages

Normal autism (birth to 2 months)

- Periods of sleep outweigh periods of arousal in a state similar to intrauterine life.

Symbiosis (2–5 months)

- Infant able to distinguish inner world from outer world as a result of developing perceptual abilities.

Differentiation (5–10 months)

- Progressive neurological development and increased alertness draw infant's attention away from self to the outer world. Physical and psychological distinctness from mother starts to form.

Practising (10–18 months)

- Child's exploration of the world increases as he/she is able to move independently.

Rapprochement (18–24 months)

- As child realizes his/her helplessness and dependence, the need for independence alternates with the need for closeness. Child moves away from his/her mother and comes back for reassurance.

Object constancy (2–5 years)

● Child gradually begins to comprehend and is reassured by the permanence of the mother and other important people, even when not in their presence.

Emotional development in infancy and childhood

Age	Emotional capacity and expression
Birth	Pleasure, surprise, disgust, distress
6–8 weeks	Joy
3–4 months	Anger
8–9 months	Sadness, fear
12–18 months	Tender affection, shame
24 months	Pride
3–4 years	Guilt, envy
5–6 years	Insecurity, humility, confidence

Kohlberg – stages of moral development

Level I: Preconventional morality – up to 10 years old

- **Stage 1:** Punishment orientation – rules are obeyed to avoid punishment.
- **Stage 2:** Reward orientation – rules are obeyed in order to obtain rewards.

Level II: Conventional morality

- **Stage 3:** Interpersonal relations – conforms to rules/expectations of family/friends to avoid disapproval by others.
- **Stage 4:** Respect for authority and social order – authority is obeyed in order to avoid feelings of guilt and to uphold social order.

Kohlberg – stages of moral development (cont.)

Level III: Postconventional morality

- **Stage 5:** Social contract orientation – upholds principles agreed as essential for society to function whilst still recognizing that different people have different views and laws can be changed.
- **Stage 6:** Universal/ethical priniciple orientation – justice is valued above rules, so there is a recognition of universal principles respecting the rights of all individuals based on values, equality, dignity and justice. Rules are obeyed to avoid self-condemnation.

Jean Piaget – characteristics achieved at each stage

Sensorimotor (birth to 2 years)
- **Object permanence:** Ability to understand that objects have an existence beyond the child's involvement with the object, so when child leaves room understands even though he/she can no longer see the object, eg chair, it is still in the room.
- **Symbolization:** Infants are able to create a visual image of an object such as a ball to stand for a real object.

Preoperational thought (2–7 years)
- **Symbolic thinking:** Concepts are primitive and children at this stage are unable to think logically.
- **Immanent justice:** They believe that punishment for bad behaviour is inevitable (rules are inviolate).
- **Egocentric:** Unable to understand others' points of views, they see themselves as the centre of the universe.
- **Phenomenalistic causality:** Events that occur together are thought to be interconnected, eg bad thoughts causing a catastrophic event.
- **Animistic thinking:** Tendency to endow physical objects and events with psychological attributes such as feelings and intentions.

Jean Piaget – characteristics achieved at each stage

Concrete operational stage (7–11 years)

- **Operational thought:** Replaces egocentric thought – children are now able to see things from someone else's perspective.
- **Syllogistic reasoning:** Logical conclusions are formed from two premises.
- **Conservation:** The ability to recognize that although the shape of some objects may change, the volume does not change and it is the same object, eg ball of clay rolled out is still same mass but in a different form.
- **Reversibility:** Capacity to understand the relationship between two different things and that one thing can turn into another and back again.

Formal operational stage (11 years to puberty)

- **Logical thinking:** Children are able to think in a highly logical and abstract manner.
- **Hypotheticodeductive reasoning:** The highest organization of cognition – allows a person to make a hypothesis and test it against reality.

Kubler Ross – stages of adaptation to death of a loved one or knowledge of facing death (terminal diagnosis)

- **Denial:** Initially the death of a loved one (or other traumatic news, eg being told about a terminal illness) is not accepted.
- **Anger:** The individual expresses anger towards family and/or friends.
- **Bargaining:** The individual starts to try to think about the death.
- **Depression:** The individual grieves openly and shares their feelings with family/friends.
- **Acceptance:** A sense of stillness and detachment replace the previous feelings.

In reality, these stages rarely take place in the order listed and may present in a different order from one individual to another.

Harlow and Lorenz – early social development

● In the 1950s and 1960s **Harlow** conducted a series of experiments exploring attachment behaviour. He tested whether food or physical closeness and contact was more important in forming an attachment. Baby rhesus monkeys preferred contact with an artificial cloth mother over feeding from another artificial object which provided food. Rhesus monkeys raised with such an artificial mother experienced a great deal of distress when separated from the surrogate mother. Monkeys who had been raised without a real mother went on to become unable to provide adequate mothering themselves and became withdrawn and unable to relate to their peers (a state similar to depression in adult humans).

● **Lorenz** believed that all animals including humans are biologically predisposed towards attachment formation. In some animals, attachment is based on 'imprinting' and becomes irreversible – the first contact that a newly hatched gosling had became ingrained in its mind and it was programmed to follow it. The first contact was usually the mother so the newborn would follow the mother. If something/someone else replaced the mother, the gosling would continue to follow that object as if it were the mother. It is felt to be an important concept in psychiatry in terms of understanding how early developmental experiences affect an individual later on in life. Lorenz also studied aggression and found that it served a practical function in animals in terms of territorial defence. Lorenz tried to apply his theories to human aggression, seeing it as serving the purpose of seeking out the best territory, necessary both early in human evolution and, to some extent, today.

Maslow's hierarchy of needs

- Maslow used previous work on factors associated with motivation in order to produce what he described as a hierarchy of needs. Prior to Maslow's work, most theorists had considered aspects of motivation separately such as biological factors, achievement, etc. Maslow attempted to integrate these factors together in his model.

- Candidates are expected to know the order of needs according to Maslow's model:

  Stage 1—Physiological/physical: Hunger, thirst, sex, food, shelter, warmth.

  Stage 2—Safety: A sense of security and proection from danger.

  Stage 3—Social belonging/love: Affiliation with others (family/friends/relationships).

  Stage 4—Self-esteem: Social acceptance, independence.

  Stage 5—Self-actualization: The highest order of need in the model and represents the stage at which the person achieves a sense of inner fulfilment and realization of personal potential.

Maslow's hierarchy of needs

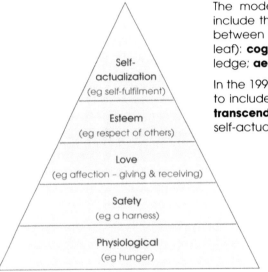

The model was adapted in the 1970s to include the following stages that would fall between stages 4 and 5 (described overleaf): **cognitive** – understanding and knowledge; **aesthetic** – order and symmetry.

In the 1990s the model was further adapted to include the last and final stage of – **self-transcendence** – helping others achieve self-actualization.

Attachment theory (developed by John Bowlby (1907–90)

Four phases of attachment

- **Indiscriminate responsiveness (0–3 months):** Young babies respond in similar ways to different people.
- **Focusing on familiar people (3–6 months):** Babies begin to respond selectively to certain people, especially main carer.
- **Intense attachment and proximity seeking (6 months to 3 years):** Intense attachment to main carer develops, associated with separation anxiety and stranger fear.
- **Partnership behaviour (3 years to adulthood):** Increasing awareness of carer's actions, and allows carer to leave.

Bowlby described separation leading to:

Protest → Despair → Detachment

Mary Ainsworth has described four types of attachment:

- **Secure attachments:** Babies use mothers as base for exploration.
- **Insecure-avoidant:** Appear to be independent, do not check for presence of mother.
- **Insecure-ambivalent:** Cling to mother, avoid exploration.
- **Disorganized:** No discernible pattern of behaviour.

Drugs affecting seizure threshold with ECT treatment

Increase seizure threshold

- Benzodiazepines.
- Anticonvulsants.
- Barbiturates.

Decrease seizure threshold

- Tricyclic antidepressants.
- Lithium.
- Antipsychotics.

Hyponatraemia induced by antidepressants

Risk factors

- Old age.
- Female.
- Low weight.
- Other drugs – NSAIDs, diuretics.
- Impaired renal function.
- Medical comorbidity.
- Warm climate.

Symptoms/signs

- Dizziness.
- Nausea.
- Lethargy.
- Confusion.
- Cramps.
- Seizures.

Management

- Stop antidepressant.
- If Na >125 monitor U&Es daily, if Na <125 refer for urgent medical management.
- When restarting treatment, consider a noradrenergic drug such as reboxetine, or ECT. Consider fluid restriction.

General facts about the DSM IV

- DSM IV can have more than one diagnosis on each axis.
- However it does not require a diagnosis on every axis.
- There is a score for the lowest recent functioning level.
- It is published in English alone; the ICD10 is published in several languages.
- DSM IV is atheoretical - it does not look at causes or pathology.

General facts about the ICD10

- It does not have a category for culture bound syndromes.
- It has a category for organic mental disorders.
- There is no section for social functioning.
- It describes disorders for both adults and children.

8. Miscellaneous topics – classification in psychiatry

ICD10 and DSM IV classifications

Comparing and contrasting

- Neurosis is not a category in ICD10 or DSM IV.
- ICD10 does not distinguish between psychosis and neurosis.
- DSM IV has its own category for psychoses.
- DSM IV is not based on research in clinical trials.
- The diagnosis of schizophrenia using ICD10 is reliable.

ICD10 and DSM IV classifications (cont.)

Comparing and contrasting (cont.)

- Reliability and validity in classifications are separate concepts.
- Having an international consensus does make classification more reliable.
- Psychiatric classification is not based on outcome.
- Classification allows conditions such as mental retardation to be classified.
- Nomothetic classification does not look at individual cases, eg Diagnosis. Idiographic classification looks at the individual case as in the five axes of DSM IV.

Interview techniques

Common mistakes

- Lack of clarification.
- Accepting jargon.
- Failure to respond to non-verbal cues.
- Premature reassurance.

Types of questions

- Open-ended – suitable for the beginning of interview or topic, eg 'What is your sleep like?'
- Closed – suitable for clarification, eg 'Do you wake up early in the morning?'
- Leading – should be avoided, eg 'Do you sleep badly?'
- Multi-thematic –should be avoided, eg 'What are your sleep and appetite like?'

Interview techniques (cont.)

Facilitating techniques
- Silences – to let the patient consider reply.
- Empathic statements – eg 'That must have been very distressing for you'.
- Respond to non-verbal cues – eg 'It seems to be upsetting for you to talk about your mother'.
- Summarizing – eg 'So far you have told me three reasons why you are depressed'.

When using an interpreter
- If possible always use trained interpreters, only use relative/friend if absolutely essential.
- Arrange seating in a triangle.
- Address patient directly and in the second person.
- Be seen to listen and respond non-verbally to patient's replies.
- Especially important to summarize.

Culture bound syndromes

- **Koro:** A fear that the genitals will shrink into the abdomen and that death will occur. It is seen in South-east Asia especially in Chinese Malaysians and in parts of China.

- **Amok**: This is found in men in Indonesia and Malaysians, and after a period of brooding there may be violence and aggression. There may be amnesia afterwards.

- **Latah:** More common in women in Malaysia and North Africa. There may be echolalia, echopraxia and automatic obedience. It is thought to be a dissociative state.

- **Dhat:** An Asian psychosexual disorder found often in Sri Lanka where loss of semen can lead to fatigue, weakness, insomnia and aches and pains.

- **Boufee delirante:** An acute stress-related psychosis which the patient often recovers from in weeks. More common in West Africa and Haiti but not limited to this subgroup. There may be psychomotor excitement and marked confusion.

Culture bound syndromes

- **Brain fag:** In West Africa male high school and university students state their brains are fatigued. There may be difficulties concentrating and symptoms of pain and pressure around the head and neck.

- **Susto:** Found in Central and South America. Anxiety and depression are attributed to the loss of soul. The individual is anxious about not being able to fulfil their role in society

- **Arctic hysteria:** Seen in Eskimo women. The individual may tear their clothes off and run about screaming. The person may be violent to others or may be at risk of hypothermia.

- **Windigo:** This is seen in North American Indians. In this depressive disorder individuals think they have mutated into a cannibalistic monster.

- **Ekbom's syndrome:** A hypochondriacal monosymptomatic psychosis.

- **Da Costa syndrome:** Another description of cardiac neurosis. The patient feels that normal signs of functioning of the heart mean something more sinister is occurring.

Common rating scales used in psychiatric assessment – observer rated vs self rated

Observer rated

- **Global assessment:** Clinical Global Impression (CGI), Global Assessment Scale (GAS), Brief Psychiatric Rating Scale (BPRS).
- **Schizophrenia:** Schedule for the Assessment of Negative Symptoms (SANS), Positive and Negative Syndrome Scale (PANS).
- **Depression:** Hamilton Depression Scale (HamD), Montgomery Asberg Depression Rating Scale (MADRS).
- **Mania:** Young Mania Rating Scale.
- **Anxiety disorders:** Hamilton Anxiety Rating Scale (HARS), Yale Brown Obsessive Compulsive Scale (YBOCS).
- **Cognitive assessment:** Mini Mental State Exam (MMSE), Cambridge Cognitive Assessment (CAMCOG), Neuropsychiatric Inventory (NPI).
- **Movement disorders:** Barnes Akathisia Rating Scale, Simpson Angus Scale for EPSEs, Abnormal Involuntary Movement Inventory (AIMS).

Common rating scales used in psychiatric assessment – observer rated vs self rated (cont.)

Self-rated

- **Depression:** Beck Depression Inventory (BDI), Zung Depression Scale, Hospital Anxiety and Depression Scale, Eating Attitudes Test (EAT), Edinburgh Postnatal Depression Scale.
- **Personality:** Minnesota Multiphasic Personality Inventory (MMPI).

Head injury

- Post-traumatic amnesia (PTA) is the time from injury until the person regains their full memory functions, particularly full episodic memory.
- Poor prognostic factors include:
  - low GCS score at time of injury
  - long duration of PTA
  - long duration of coma.
- 30% chance of epilepsy if injury was penetrating, 5% in closed head injuries.
- Executive dysfunction may occur – characterized by decreased retention in memory for new information, poor short term recall and verbal and visuospatial deficits.

Head injury (cont.)

- Depression common (around 25% post trauma up to several months although most recover).
- Mania occurs rarely.
- PTSD occurs in 10–20% of cases.
- 30% sustain personality changes such as paranoid, avoidant or impulsive characteristics. These may improve up to 2 years after the trauma.

Organic conditions associated with psychiatric symptoms

Neurological

- Cerebrovascular disorders (haemorrhage, infection).
- Head trauma (concussion, post-traumatic haematoma).
- Narcolepsy.
- Brain neoplasms.
- Normal pressure hydrocephalus.
- Parkinson's disease.
- Multiple sclerosis.
- Huntington's disease.
- Alzheimer's dementia.
- Metachromatic leukodystrophy.
- Migraine.

Organic conditions associated with psychiatric symptoms (cont.)

Endocrine
- Hypo/hyperthyroidism/adrenalism/parathyroidism/ glycaemia.
- Diabetes mellitus.
- Panhypopituitarism.
- Phaeochromocytoma.
- Pregnancy.
- Gonadotrophic hormonal disturbances.

Metabolic/ nutritional
- Electrolyte imbalance (eg syndrome of inappropriate secretion of ADH (SIADH)).
- Hypotension.
- Hypoxaemia.
- Hypertensive encephalopathy.
- Porphyria.
- Uraemia.
- Wilson's disease (hepatolenticular degeneration).
- Hepatic encephalopathy.
- Deficiency of vitamin B_{12}, nicotinic acid, folate, thiamine, magnesium or zinc.
- Malnutrition/dehydration.

Organic conditions associated with psychiatric symptoms

Toxic

- Intoxication or withdrawal from a substance.
- Adverse effects of some non-psychiatric medications.
- Environmental toxins (eg heavy metals, organophosphates).

Infectious

- AIDS.
- Neurosyphilis.
- Viral meningitis/encephalitis.
- Brain abscess.
- Tuberculosis.
- Streptococcal infections.
- Viral hepatitis.
- Infectious mononucleosis.
- Systemic bacterial or viral infections.

Organic conditions associated with psychiatric symptoms

Autoimmune

- Systemic lupus erythematosus (SLE).

Neoplastic

- CNS primary and metastatic tumours.
- Endocrine tumours.
- Pancreatic carcinoma.
- Paraneoplastic syndromes.

Mnemonic – INMATE

I = Infectious.
N = Neoplastic.
M = Metabolic.
A = Autoimmune.
T = Tumours.
E = Endocrine.

Reasons why people fail an explanation station

- Conducting a monologue without adequately allowing the patient to talk and ask questions.

- Not answering a patient's question. This is a common pitfall. Nobody knows everything. If you don't know the answer to a question, then say so. Say you will find the answer and let them know next time you meet with them. Don't just avoid the question.

- There is a common misconception among candidates that they must explain every aspect of a diagnosis as if answering an essay. If you do not get to say everything you wanted in the time given, then tell the patient, and say you would like to arrange to meet them again, just as you would in clinical practice.

Reasons why people fail an assessment station

● Missing key aspects of the assessment – try to always touch on the following aspects of history in any assessment:
—History of mood disturbance/suicidality.
—History of psychotic symptoms.
—History of drug or alcohol misuse.
—Risk assessment.
For example, if asked to assess for postnatal depression all of the above are relevant.

● Missing several key aspects of the history relevant to a specific station – for example if asked to assess premorbid personality, the candidate should cover a reasonable number of the points on OSCE 2 (card 107). The candidate should strike a balance between asking relevant questions whilst still engaging and listening to the patient. If the candidate focuses solely on 'the right set of questions' and doesn't take the time to listen to the patient, s/he is likely to fail that station.

Scenario

A patient is admitted to your ward and has strange beliefs that the government has been conducting experiments on him since the 1960s. He believes that they are responsible for his recent hernia operation.

Interview in order to elicit delusions

Suggested approach

1. Good communication
2. Probe broadly for presence of different types of delusions
3. Enquire about comorbidity
4. Risk assessment

1. Good communication – Introduce yourself and approach the topic with tact.

2. Probe broadly for the presence of delusions –
- Ask about delusions of persecution. In this case the government may feature strongly.
- Ask about delusions of reference and delusional misinterpretation.
- Enquire about delusions of guilt.
- Enquire about grandiose delusions.
- Ask about nihilistic delusions and hypochondriasis.
- Delusional jealousy is important owing to its potentially disastrous consequences.
- Religious delusions.
- Delusional mood and passivity phenomena.
- Establish whether delusions are primary or secondary.
- The fixity of the beliefs must be gauged – are these true delusions?
- Try to find out the extent of systematization of the belief system. Are the delusions encapsulated?

3. Ask about comorbidity – Alcohol or substance misuse, depressive symptoms and briefly screen for other psychotic symptoms.

4. Risk assessment – Find out whether the patient has acted on the delusions and harmed himself or others. Do they cause distress to the patient?

Scenario

A 46-year-old man is on the drug and alcohol rehabilitation ward undergoing alcohol detoxification. He became depressed after his wife died 11 years ago in a car accident. He began drinking heavily and subsequently lost his job and has suffered depression ever since. He is currently unemployed and on incapacity benefit. He is undergoing alcohol detoxification and says he wants to try to 'get his life back again'.

Take a history to establish his premorbid personality

Suggested approach

1. Good communication
2. Ask about features of premorbid personality

1. Good communication – Introduce yourself and explain your role. Say you would like to ask a few questions to find about the patients personality prior to the death of his wife and before be became depressed.

2. Ask about features of premorbid personality: mnemonic – MRI DOC FIBS

M - Mood – How did you used to feel in yourself as a person? Would you describe yourself as a happy person? Or have you always tended to worry about things?

R - Relationships – How many relationships did you have before you became unwell? Were there any difficulties? Do you feel that there were any aspects of your personality that contributed to the problems?

I - Interests – What things did you used to enjoy doing in your spare time?

D - Drugs – Had you ever used any drugs before you became unwell for the first time?

O - Obsessions or compulsions – Have you ever been very particular about details? Do you feel the need to check doors are locked or do you worry a lot about hygiene?

C - Coping strategies – How did you used to deal with problems?

F - Fantasy life – Before you became unwell, did you used to have any plans or ambitions for the future? Did you used to fantasize about anything?

I - Impulsivity – Did you ever use to do things on the spur of the moment that you later regretted?

B - Beliefs – Were you a religious person? Do you believe in anything?

S - Sexuality – What is your sexual orientation?

Scenario

A 22-year-old man has been admitted to hospital for the second time, after airport staff raised concerns about him lying on the seats and 'acting funny' looking suspicious and asking about 'the radio waves'. On admission, he told you that the planes were sending out radio waves to him and he could control their flight path with these waves. Over the last 2 months it seems likely from your assessments that he has a diagnosis of schizophrenia as all other possibilities are ruled out. His mother already has an inkling that this might be his diagnosis, and she wants to know more about it.

1. Explain to his mother what a diagnosis of schizophrenia means.
2. Address any concerns the mother may have

Suggested approach to any 'Explain a diagnosis' station

1. Good communication
2. Explain the nature of the illness
3. Explain what factors are thought to lead to the illness
4. Explain the likely course and prognosis
5. Explain key treatments available

Make sure you link your explanation to the patient's symptoms. Don't just give a textbook answer.

1. Good communication: I'd like to explain a bit about this illness called schizophrenia to you, but before I start, do you have any particular questions or concerns? Do you know anything already about this illness?

2. Explain the nature of the illness: Schizophrenia is a common condition that affects about 1 in every 100 people. Normally, there is a link between the way we think, our emotions and behaviour, and the way we perceive things with our hearing and other senses. In schizophrenia, that normal link is lost, so that thoughts, feelings, behaviour and perception can change. What that means is that people might hear or see things that aren't there. Or they might have odd thoughts like feeling paranoid about other people or like when your son thought he could control the aeroplanes.

3. Explain what factors are thought to lead to the illness: No exact cause found. Can run in families – first degree relative has a 10-fold higher chance of developing the illness. Complications at birth may be a factor in affecting neurodevelopment which may be a risk factor for developing schizophrenia. Stress can act as a trigger to onset or relapse. Stress alone may not be a direct cause. Marijuana has been shown to be associated with a greater chance of developing schizophrenia.

4. Explain the likely course and prognosis: Can be lifelong/relapsing remitting/chronic. Explain there is reason to be hopeful and be optimistic.

5. Explain key treatments available: Antipsychotic drugs – correct the chemical imbalance. Psychological input – CBT to provide coping strategies/distraction techniques and to challenge delusional beliefs. Support from: the Community Mental Health Team; Social Support; OT input to assess Activities of Daily Living.

Scenario

You are asked to see a 56-year-old lady as a liaison referral on the medical ward. She was diagnosed with leukaemia 6 years ago and was admitted yesterday following a relapse of her symptoms. The medical SHO has asked you to see her as she appears somewhat depressed.

Enquire about her mood

Suggested approach

1. Good communication
2. Assess for depressive symptoms
3. Ask about comorbidity
4. Perform a thorough risk assessment

1. Good communication – Introduce yourself and explain your role as the junior psychiatrist. Take a sensitive approach. Try to speak at the same volume as the patient and lean forwards as you talk to her. As she talks about her leukaemia show empathy by saying 'I'm sorry to hear that, it sounds as if you have been going through a very difficult time'. Ask open questions to begin with – 'How have you been feeling lately?' and then 'can you tell me a bit more about what you've been going through that has lead to you feeling depressed?'

2. Assess for depressive symptoms. Ask about – mnemonic: EMI CEG PASS

E – Energy (loss of).
M – Mood (pervasive low mood on most days over at least 2 weeks).
I – Interest (loss of interest in activities – anhedonia).
C – Concentration (poor).
E – Esteem (low self esteem).
G – Guilt (feelings of guilt).
P – Pessimism (feelings of hopelessness).
A – Appetite (poor or excessive).
S – Sleep (disturbance, early morning wakening).
S – Suicidal thoughts.
For an ICD10 diagnosis of:
Mild depressive episode – need 2 from EMI and 2 from CEG PASS.
Moderate depressive episode – need 2 from EMI and 3 from CEG PASS.
Severe depressive episode – all 3 from EMI and 4 from CEG PASS, one of which must include suicidal thoughts. Severe depressive episode can be +/– psychotic symptoms which are usually mood congruent delusions or hallucinations.

3. Ask about comorbidity – Ask about psychotic symptoms and substance misuse.

4. Perform a thorough risk assessment – Enquire tactfully about suicidal thoughts. First say 'I'm sorry to hear that you've been going through a difficult time. Sometimes do you ever feel as if life is not worth living any more or as if you wish you wouldn't wake up in the morning?' Then if they say yes, ask, 'Do you ever have any thoughts of ending your life'. Then go on to ask about specific suicidal ideas and their extent and if any suicidal plans have been made.

Scenario

You have been asked to see a 28-year-old lady who has self-presented to the A&E department with acute chest pain and shortness of breath. This is her second presentation in the past week. The medical senior house officer has excluded an organic cause for her symptoms and believes there may be a psychological cause.

Take a history focusing on symptoms of anxiety, in order to formulate a diagnosis

Suggested approach

1. Good communication
2. Elicit symptoms to differentiate between different anxiety disorders
3. Ask about panic attacks
4. Ask about avoidance behaviour
5. Ask about comorbidity
6. Explore impact on life and risk assessment

1. Good communication – 'Hello, I am Dr. Patel. I am one of the junior psychiatrists here today. I have been asked to see you to talk about the chest pain you have been experiencing recently to see if there is anything we can do to help. Would that be OK? Can you tell me what has been happening recently?' – Now allow the patient to talk. Comment on non-verbal and verbal cues, eg if the patient dips her head as she talks about the recent death of her father, say 'that sounds very sad'.

2. Elicit symptoms to differentiate between different anxiety disorders – Symptoms: onset/duration/precipitants/frequency. **Psychological symptoms:** apprehension, worry, nervousness, fear of fainting, vomiting, going mad or dying. **Physical symptoms:** palpitations, rapid heart rate, sweating, breathlessness, tremor. **Circumstances in which symptoms occur:** differentiate between agoraphobia, social phobia, specific phobias and generalized anxiety disorder (GAD). **Agoraphobia:** fear of leaving the safety of the home, fear of travelling alone. **Social phobia:** fear of embarrassment, fear of small group situations. **Specific phobia:** fear of a specific object, fear of a specific place. **GAD:** excessive worry about the future, feeling tense and nervous all the time.

3. Ask about panic attack symptoms – Do you feel as if you are choking/fainting/about to die when these attacks occur.

4. Ask about avoidance behaviour – Anything done to avoid these attacks?

5. Screen for associated mood/psychotic symptoms and ask about substance misuse.

6. Ask about impact on life and risk assessment – Effect on family/friends/partners/work/self-care/care of children or other dependents. Ask about any suicidal thoughts.

Scenario

You are the SHO working in the Old Age Psychiatry Team. A 67-year-old man is referred to you by his GP as he has been complaining that he has been experiencing memory problems over the last few months. He says sometimes he will leave his keys on the kitchen top and then forgets where he left them. He then feels disorientated at times trying to remember their location.

Perform a cognitive examination

Suggested approach

1. Good communication
2. Assess orientation, concentration and short term recall
3. Assess memory – intermediate and long term
4. Assess frontal, parietal and temporal lobes

1. Good communication – Introduce and explain your role. Explain that you would like to test his memory and some other aspects of his brain function with some simple tests.

2. Orientation – Day/date/month/year/season. Place – country/county/town/building/floor. **Registration** – Ask to say an address, eg James Smith, 59 Penn Street, Victoria, London. **Attention/concentration** – Spell the word WORLD. Then backwards. **Recall** – ask to recall address given earlier.

3. Memory – Recent (intermediate term) – What did you do yesterday evening?/Long term – What was your address where you grew up as a child?

4. Frontal lobe assessment – (i) History of incontinence, change in smell (?inferior lesion), visual changes (?homonymous hemianopia), change in affect/behaviour eg becoming disinhibited. (ii) Verbal fluency: name as many words as possible beginning with S in one minute. (iii) Luria Motor Test. (iv) Cognitive estimates: how tall is a bus? Or assess proverb interpretation. (v) Listen for verbal perseveration. (vi) Reflexes: palmomental and grasp. (vii) Assess gait (viii) Tapping test: response inhibition or check for utilization behaviour.

5. Parietal lobe assessment – (i) Speech: repetition, naming (?nominal dysphasia), fluency – (?receptive/expressive dysphasia). (ii) Right-left disorientation and sensory inattention: three-stage command (ask to take paper in left hand, fold in half and return with right hand). (iii) Assess for Constructional/Dressing apraxia (iv) Astereognosia: ask to recognize common object placed in hand with eyes closed. (v) Agraphasthesia: ask to recognize letter drawn on palm of hand. (vi) Writing.

6. Temporal lobe assessment – False thinking, jamais vu/déjà vu experiences, panoramic memory, hallucinations, gastric sensations, motor seizures (lip smacking/involuntary movements).

Scenario

A 26-year-old lady presents to A&E in an intoxicated state. You are asked to assess her by the A&E doctor as she is sober now and saying she has been feeling depressed and drinking heavily over the last few weeks since her boyfriend left her.

Take a history to elicit symptoms of alcohol dependency

Suggested approach

1. Good communication
2. Enquire about alcohol use
3. Establish features of dependency
4. Ask about comorbidity
5. Explore impact on functioning and risk assessment

1. Good communication – Introduce yourself and explain your role as a junior psychiatrist. Say you would like to ask a few questions about her alcohol use and ask if that would be OK. Start with open questions, eg 'can you please tell me what has been happening?' Then move on to more closed questions.

2. Enquire about alcohol use – Onset, frequency, duration and drinking behaviour (types of drinks, sources, how the habit is being financed).

3. Establish features of dependency – ICD10 Criteria: three or more of the following are required to establish a syndrome of dependency to any psychoactive substance including alcohol – **mnemonic** – **CCST WU**

C – Compulsion (a strong desire to use alcohol).
C – Control (difficulty controlling use in terms of onset, stopping, levels of use).
S – Salience (progressive neglect of alternative pleasures or interests due to alcohol use, increased amount of time necessary to obtain or take the substance or recover from its effects, ie alcohol takes over one's life).
T – Tolerance: increasing doses are required to produce the same effects as were previously present with lower doses.
W – Withdrawal: physiological state of withdrawal may present with sweating, insomnia, tachycardia, nausea or vomiting, grand mal seizures, delirium tremens.
U – Use despite harmful effects.

Alternatively candidates may prefer to remember the criteria for alcohol dependency described by Edwards and Gross: (i) Narrowing of the drinking repertoire. (ii) Drink-seeking behaviour. (iii) Tolerance. (iv) Withdrawal. (v) Drinking to relieve or avoid withdrawal symptoms. (vi) Subjective awareness of the compulsion to drink. (vii) Rapid reinstatement of drinking after a period of abstinence.

4. Ask about comorbidity – Enquire about depression, psychotic symptoms or other substance misuse.

5. Risk assessment – Enquire about physical risk issues: poor diet/malnutrition, liver disease (may need to be referred to a physician). Ask if there have been any suicidal thoughts, ideas or plans or any thoughts of harming others.

Scenario

A 32-year-old man is referred to your outpatient clinic by his GP. He describes a history of several difficult relationships since he was 16 years old when he had his first partner. He says he feels extremely depressed when the relationships end and sometimes feels suicidal. He often cuts himself superficially on his forearms and once took an overdose.

Take a history to establish if he has features of emotionally unstable personality disorder – borderline type

Suggested approach

1. Good communication
2. Enquire about features of borderline personality disorder
3. Ask about comorbidity
4. Risk assessment

1. Good communication – Introduce and explain your role (eg 'Hello I am Dr. Smith, I am a junior psychiatrist, I have come to ask you a few questions about your personality. Knowing about your personality could be useful to us in understanding you better so that we can try to help you as best as we can, would that be OK?').

2. Enquire about features of borderline personality disorder. ICD10 Diagnosis – mnemonic: DEARS

D - **D**isturbed self-image: the patient's own image, aims and internal preferences are often unclear or disturbed.

E - **E**motional instability: a tendency to act impulsively without consideration of the consequences and chronic feelings of **E**mptiness.

A - **A**ffective instability and feelings of **A**bandonment.

R - **R**elationship difficulties: a tendency to become involved in intense and unstable relationships leading to repeated emotional crises and may be associated with excessive efforts to avoid abandonment.

S - **S**uicidal threats and **S**elf-harming behaviour: often associated with relationship difficulties but may occur separately as well.

3. Ask about comorbidity – Enquire if the patient has felt depressed or experienced any psychotic symptoms (which may be a feature of personality disorders) and if they have been using any illicit drugs.

4. Risk assessment - Enquire about suicidal thoughts, ideas or plans as well if there has been any self-cutting or other self-injurious behaviour. Ask if there are any thoughts of harming others.

Scenario

A 48-year-old man has been admitted on to the ward. He has a history of offending behaviour since adolescence and has been charged in the past for burglary as well as grievous bodily harm for which he served 2 years in prison. He has a history of attendance at a child psychiatric service when he was 14 years old due to bad behaviour at school – bullying other children and destroying property. He has suffered from depression with associated polysubstance misuse over the past 20 years and has now been admitted after taking an overdose of some analgesic tablets.

Take a history with a view to establishing a diagnosis of dissocial (antisocial) personality disorder

Suggested approach

1. Good communication
2. Ask about features of dissocial personality disorder
3. Enquire about comorbidity
4. Risk assessment

1. Good communication – Introduce and explain your role (eg 'Hello I am Dr Smith, I am a junior psychiatrist, I have come to ask you a few questions about your personality. Knowing about your personality could be useful to us in understanding you better so that we can try to help you as best as we can, would that be OK?').

2. Enquire about features of dissocial personality disorder. ICD 10 criteria – mnemonic: FIGURE

F – Frustration (low tolerance to frustration and a low threshold for discharge of aggression).

I – Irresponsibility (gross and persistent attitude of irresponsibility and disregard for social norms, rules and obligations).

G – Guilt (incapacity to experience guilt or to profit from experience, particularly punishment).

U – Unconcern for the feelings of others (callous unconcern).

R – Relationship difficulties (incapacity to maintain enduring relationships, though having no difficulty in establishing them).

E – Externalize blame (blames others or offers plausible rationalizations for behaviour which has brought the individual into conflict with society).

3. Enquire about comorbidity – Ask about depression, pychotic symptoms and substance misuse.

4. Risk assessment – Ask about a history of offending behaviour including any charges or convictions and sentences. Ask if there are any current thoughts of self-harm or anyone the person is currently at odds with and if there are any thoughts of harming others.

Scenario

A 55-year-old lady who suffers from schizophrenia has come to see you in your out-patient clinic. She has been treated with chlorpromazine over the last 13 years. You notice that her arms appear to be shaking somewhat.

Assess the patient for extrapyramidal side effects

Suggested approach

1. Good communication
2. History of extrapyramidal symptoms
3. General observation
4. General examination
5. Assess gait

1.Good communication

'Hello, I am Dr X. I am one of the junior psychiatrists. I've been asked to examine you for possible side-effects of your medication. Would that be all right with you?'

'I notice that your arms are shaking. This may be a side-effect of the medication that you're taking. Would you mind if I check for other possible effects that the medication could be having?'

'Would you mind if I ask a female nurse to join us?'

2. History of extrapyramidal symptoms
'Have you noticed that your arms are shaking?'
'Does it trouble you? How long has it been going on?'
'Has anyone changed the dose of your tablets at any point in time?'
'Do you wear dentures?'
'Have you noticed any movements of your tongue, lips or mouth that you can't control?'
'Do you ever feel restless?'
'Have you noticed any stiffness or aching in your muscles?'
'Do you grind your teeth at night?'

3. General observation – comment on:
- Facial expression and evidence of oral-mandibular-lingual signs: chewing movements, rabbit syndrome, bon bon sign, grimacing, pouting, repetitive swallowing, trismus, mask-like facies.
- Signs of akathisia: legs shaking.
- Parkinsonian tremor: resting tremor.
- Limb movements: such as ballismus.
- Neck/spine signs: torticollis, antecollis, retrocollis, pleurothotonus, opisthotonus, axial hyper-kinesias.
- Ocular signs: blepharospasm, oculogyric crisis.
- Vocal tics, dysphonia (from vocal cord spasm), stridor.
- Look for drooling, which may result from increased salivation and dysphagia.

Note that a resting tremor is made worse by anxiety and is improved by voluntary movement.
A common mistake is for candidates to check resting tremor by asking patients to put their arms out; this is incorrect. Ask the patient to rest their hands on their legs – this is the correct position.

4. General examination

● Start with the arms: look for a 'pill-rolling' resting tremor and then check tone. There may be lead-pipe rigidity and, if tremor is superimposed, cogwheel rigidity.

● Next do a glabellar tap. To do this, repeatedly tap the patient's mid-forehead between the eyebrows with the tip of your finger. In people experiencing parkinsonian side-effects, the patient may demonstrate a glabellar tap sign, in which he/she continues to blink. False positives are fairly common, however.

● Examine the tongue. Ask the patient to stick out the tongue for a few seconds. Look for any fasciculation

● Posture. Ask the patient to stand. Observe whether he/she is stooped (parkinsonian).

● Check for truncal stability. Slightly nudge the patient forwards and backwards and from side to side. In parkinsonism there is a tendency for the patient to lose their balance because of slow correcting movements.

● Check the limbs for cogwheel rigidity

● Lastly ask the patient to write a sentence. Observe for micrographia.

5. Assess gait

● Ask the patient to walk from one end of the room to the other.

● Observe the arm swing. In parkinsonism the arms do not swing fully.

● Parkinsonian gait – toe walking, slow, stooped gait. In parkinsonism the gait may be shuffling and the patient may show festination.

Scenario

A 26-year-old receptionist has recently been admitted to hospital for the first time in a manic state. The consultant tells you in the ward round that she should be started on Lithium therapy.

Explain lithium treatment to the patient.

Suggested Approach to any 'Explain a treatment' station –

1. **Good Communication**
2. **Explain the nature of the treatment (what it is, how it works, indications)**
3. **Explain its benefits**
4. **Explain potential side effects/ negative consequences**
5. **Explain practical aspects (e.g. blood tests needed)**

Make sure you link your explanation to the patient's history.
Don't just give a textbook answer.

Points to include

1. Good communication –

Introduce yourself and explain your role as a junior psychiatrist
Establish rapport and do not include jargon. You don't have to include all the facts; good communication style is the key!
Ask the patient what they understand about their illness. Ask whether they have heard about Lithium and whether they have any particular concerns with the medication.

2. Explain the nature of the treatment –
Explain that Lithium is a mood stabiliser, which is effective in treatment of mania, hypomania or bipolar affective disorder, as well as depression that is refractory to other medications.

3. Explain benefits –
Lithium has been used widely and well established in psychiatry over the last few decades. It has been very effective in treating bipolar affective disorder and it may reduce the frequency and severity of depressive episodes.

4. Explain side effects –
Common side effects as well as symptoms/signs of toxicity should be explained (described on card 56). Explain that lithium has to be maintained at the correct level in the blood, otherwise there is a risk of toxicity. Explain that side effects can be more likely when starting some other medications, when the weather is hot or when sweating a lot as blood lithium levels may become elevated. They can also occur with certain physical health problems such as diarrhoea. Explain that if experiencing increased tremor, unsteadiness, slurred speech, double vision, producing less urine or experiencing fits or confusion to contact the GP or NHS direct immediately. Longer term risks include developing an under active thyroid (hypothyroidism), heart (ECG) changes, exacerbations of psoriasis and possible kidney changes.

5. Explain practical points – Blood tests initially at baseline including thyroid function, renal function, urea and electrolytes. A baseline ECG will also be required. Blood will be tested weekly until the correct plasma level is reached, then every 3-6 months. Ask if the patient is planning to get pregnant and explain that they will need to tell the team in advance if this is the case. If asked, risks to the unborn include Ebstein's anomaly. The patient may wish to stop Lithium before conception and restart in the 3rd trimester. Breast feeding should not be performed when taking Lithium. If Lithium is stopped altogether, there is a high chance (50%) of relapse especially after child birth.

Scenario

You have been asked to assess a 70-year-old man who has developed gangrene in his right foot. The surgical team are ready to amputate his foot as the gangrene may spread and threaten the patient's life. The patient is currently refusing surgery.

Assess the patient's capacity in relation to his decision to refuse treatment.

Suggested approach

1. Good communication
2. Assess patient's understanding of the nature of the treatment/procedure being offered. Assess reasons for refusing treatment
3. Assess the ability of the patient to retain the information given
4. Assess patient's ability to understand the benefits of having the procedure as well as the potential consequences of not having the procedure and his ability to weigh these factors in the balance
5. Assess for psychiatric symptoms that are of a nature which impair the patient's ability to make rational decisions

1. Good communication – It is often useful in practice to speak to the surgical team to clarify facts, you may not get this opportunity in the OSCE station. It is not your job to coerce, convince or persuade the patient to go through with the treatment or procedure; this is a common mistake among exam candidates. Ask about the patient's understanding of the problems (gangrene) and what the surgeons have told him about the gangrene. Ask whether he has had any operations before and if he has had a bad experience or knows anyone who had a similar experience.

2. Assess the patient's understanding of the nature of the procedure and reasons for refusing treatment – Ask about the patient's understanding of practical points – how long the procedure takes and risks associated with it. If the patient appears unclear, do not try to explain the procedure yourself (this is the surgeon's role).

3. Assess the ability of the patient to retain the information given – Assess the patient's orientation to time, place and person and their immediate, short term and long term memory. If there is a comorbid alcohol dependency or dementia, a full cognitive assessment including frontal/parietal and temporal lobe exam may be necessary, which you could say you would arrange at another time.

4. Assess patient's ability to understand the benefits of having the procedure as well as potential consequences of not having the procedure and his ability to weigh these factors in the balance – Assess the patient's understanding of how the procedure will benefit him and his knowledge of the consequences of not having the procedure. Assess broadly his ability to be able to rationally weigh these factors in the balance.

5. Assess for psychiatric symptoms that are of a nature which impair the patient's ability to make rational decisions – Ask screening questions to search for psychiatric symptoms that specifically impair the patient's ability to make a rational decision (eg delusions that the surgeons have been sent by someone to chop his foot off). Note: Simply being depressed or psychotic does not mean the patient lacks capacity.

Scenario

A 67-year-old man has been admitted to hospital after a transient ischaemic attack (TIA). This is the third time he has had a TIA. You are asked to see the patient, who is experiencing memory difficulties and appears confused, on the medical ward. You are unable to gain a history from the husband as he appears confused and does not answer questions clearly. His wife is present on the ward however.

Speak to his wife to gain a collateral history about her husband

Suggested approach

1. Good communication
2. Explore widely the nature and course of the symptoms experienced, focusing on features suggestive of vascular dementia
3. Ask about associated comorbidity – physical/psychiatric illnesses
4. Explore overall impact on functioning
5. Perform a risk assessment

1. Good communication – Introduce and explain your role. Verify that this is the wife of the patient. Ask open questions to begin such as what changes she has noticed in her husband.

2. Explore widely the nature and course of the symptoms experienced, focusing on features suggestive of vascular dementia – Ask about the time course of the symptoms and whether there has been a stepwise or gradual decline. Ask whether there are fluctuations in the symptoms. Ask specific questions regarding the patient's memory, confusion, personality and mood. Ask questions to try to establish if there was a temporal relationship between the TIAs and the symptoms developing. Enquire about language and executive functions. Screen for features of frontal lobe dementia including disinhibition and changes in personality.

3. Ask about associated comorbidity – Ask about risk factors including hypertension, diabetes, vascular disease, hypercholesterolaemia and previous cardiac events. Ask whether the patient has demonstrated symptoms suggestive of a psychotic or affective illness or another psychiatric problem.

4. Explore overall impact on functioning – Ask about level of functioning at home in terms of activities of daily living – self-care, etc. Ask whether she is able to cope at home and requires any support such as carers.

5. Perform a risk assessment – Assess risk including whether any appliances have been left on by accident, history of wandering or getting lost, any dangerous situations the patient has got into.

20. OSCE 14 – Explain systematic desensitization

Scenario

A patient has been referred to your outpatient clinic by her GP as she has been experiencing claustrophobia which has got to a point where it is causing her to feel depressed and affecting her life significantly on a day to day basis. You decide to offer her systematic desensitization.

Explain systematic desensitization to the patient

Suggested approach to any 'Explain a treatment' station

1. Good communication
2. Explain the nature of the treatment (what it is, how it works, indications)
3. Explain advantages (its benefits)
4. Explain disadvantages (potential negative effects)
5. Explain practical aspects (eg number of sessions etc.)

Make sure you link your explanation to the patient's history. Don't just give a text-book answer

1. Good communication - Give your name and explain who you are. Explain that you would like to offer her this treatment and ask if she has heard, read or knows anything about it already.

2. Explain the nature of the treatment/3. Explain the advantages (benefits) - Systematic desensitization is a behavioural technique that can be used to treat phobias such as claustrophobia that the patient is suffering from. It involves exposing the individual gradually to the feared situation. The patient must make a list of situations that cause anxiety – a list of about 10 (in a hierarchy) with equally graded increasing levels of anxiety. Sometimes there is more than one situation that provokes anxiety. Here the unifying fear(s) should be sought and tackled. If there is no common link two separate hierarchies can be made. The patient imagines or enters the situation while relaxing until they can do this without anxiety. Relaxation techniques can be taught at the same time. This is repeated with each item of the hierarchy.

4. Explain disadvantages (potential negative effects) - Pitfalls may include if the patient's anxiety worsens, the situation looked at in therapy actually causes more anxiety each time the patient attends a session (sensitization rather than desensitization).

5.Explain practical aspects – The sessions are usually once a week and last for about 1 hour. Usually the course is about 16-20 sessions although some patient's may require longer.

Scenario

A 44-year-old man is referred by his GP after several appointments where he has insisted that his wife is having an extramarital affair. Things have got to the stage where he has been checking her underwear on a daily basis.

Assess for features of morbid jealousy

Suggested approach

1. Good communication
2. Assess for presence of thoughts about partner's infidelity and if these thoughts are of a delusional quality or intensity
3. Assess for comorbidity
4. Comprehensive risk assessment

1. Good communication – Introduce and explain role. Approach topic sensitively and with tact. Ask open questions including what has been occurring lately.

2. Assess for presence of thoughts about partner's infidelity and assess if these are delusional in quality or intensity – Find out why he is suspicious and what evidence he has to support his beliefs. Find out whether the beliefs are held to a delusional fixity by asking if there is any possibility he may be wrong and exploring widely if there is a rational explanation for his views. Ask what he has been doing to check on his wife, including following her and invading her privacy. Enquire if the partner has ever cheated on him in the past, ie could the belief(s) be true? Ask if he has always been faithful to his wife. Take a full psychosexual history to enquire about past relationships and any difficulties. Ask about any sexual problems/impotence. Request consent to speak to the wife to ascertain her version of events as well as her views on his beliefs.

3. Assess for comorbidity – Screen for psychotic disorders, mood disorders, OCD, personality disorders and drug and especially alcohol problems. Ask about physical health problems also.

4. Comprehensive risk assessment –Ask if he sees himself as jealous and if he has ever been violent. Assess broadly the risk of him causing harm to the partner by probing adequately into depth of beliefs and searching for clues to indicate a grudge or other indicator of likely violence to the wife. Ask specifically if he has had any thoughts of hurting his wife in any way.

Scenario

You are speaking to the wife of a patient suffering from schizophrenia on the ward. The patient threatened his wife with a knife prior to the admission.

Assess the patient's risk of violence by talking to the wife.

Suggested approach

1. Good communication
2. Assess for history of violent behaviour
3. Ask about past relationship between mental state and violent behaviour if there was any
4. Risk assessment – current

1. Good communication – Remember you are talking to the wife and not the patient. Introduce and explain role. Ask open questions about previous and current history of violence either to the wife or to others and what this entailed.

2. Assess for history of violent behaviour – Ascertain whether there is a forensic history (a history of offending behaviour, criminal offences and charges/convictions).

3. Ask about past relationship between mental state and violent behaviour if there was any – Ascertain the context of the violence – whether it was during a psychotic relapse when the patient may have been poorly adherent with medication. Ask if the patient is dependent on illicit substances and if violence is associated with their use. Find out if anger management is a particular issue.

4. Risk assessment - current – Ask whether there are any children and if they have been affected. Has the patient told his wife about any command hallucinations or any cause for his violence? Ask if the patient has described persecutory delusions. Has the patient threatened to be violent towards himself with self-harm or suicide? Ask if the wife can cope with the situation and whether she has or intends to press charges.

Scenario

You see a 21-year-old girl in A&E who is complaining of depression. On further questioning she tells you she has been checking taps lately.

Assess for symptoms of obsessive-compulsive disorder

Suggested approach

1. Good communication
2. Assess for symptoms of OCD
3. Assess for associated comorbidity – depression, psychosis, substance misuse
4. Explore impact on functioning
5. Risk assessment

1. Good communication – Introduce and develop rapport. Ask open questions about the problem including timing, frequency and severity of symptoms.

2. Assess for symptoms of OCD – Ask about the nature and quality of obsessions including what they are, whether they are intrusive and what effect they have on the patient. Ask if there are images, ruminations or excessive doubts. Ask whether the thoughts are recognized as her own thoughts and if there is a resistance to the obsessive thoughts. It is important to ask whether the patient can control or neutralize the compulsions. Ask whether there is a magical quality between what the patient is doing and trying to achieve. Ask about what will happen if the compulsions are ignored (eg does the patient feel as if a disaster will occur?). Explore if there are any thoughts of contamination, aggressive thoughts, sexual or religious thoughts, concerns about preciseness/order, hoarding behaviour and any aspects of the body the patient checks or is concerned about.

3. Assess for associated comorbidity – Screen for other illnesses briefly including depression and psychotic thoughts. If extra time is available ask about OCD spectrum disorders including Tourette's disorder, body dysmorphic disorder and hypochondriasis. Ask whether the patient has resorted to drugs or alcohol as a result of the problem.

4. Explore impact on functioning – Is the patient able to perform activites of daily living, eg self-care, shopping, cooking, etc., or are their symptoms so severe that they interfere with their day to day ability to function. Gauge the patients insight into the problem.

5. Risk assessment – Ask if the patient has got into any dangerous situations as a result of their obsessions or compulsions. Enquire broadly about other aspects of risk – self-neglect may be an issue. Ask if symptoms have been so distressing that they have had suicidal thoughts.

Scenario

A 28-year-old unemployed male complains of a recent seizure and a funny feeling he has been here before.

Assess for temporal lobe epilepsy

Suggested approach

1. Good communication
2. Assess for symptoms of temporal lobe epilepsy
3. Enquire about comorbidity – psychosis, depression, substance misuse
4. Risk assessment

1. Good communication – Introduce and develop rapport. Ask open questions to begin with.

2. Assess for symptoms of temporal lobe epilepsy – Take a history of the seizure including timing, duration, eye witness accounts, whether the patient required medical attention. Establish if there have been any seizures and if so were they generalized tonic-clonic or an absence seizures? If generalized tonic-clonic seizures ask whether there was tongue biting or incontinence. Find out if there is any family history of epilepsy. Ask whether there was an aura before the seizure. Ask how the patient was after the seizure and whether he was drowsy and confused. Ask about the presence of any hallucinatory experiences including voices or musical sounds. Were there any visual distortions of colour or size and shape of objects? Enquire about déjà vu or jamais vu experiences.

3. Enquire about comorbidity – Ask about a family history of mood disorder or whether the patient has experienced affective symptoms. Summarize and answer questions.

4. Risk assessment – Ask whether the patient became violent at any point while he had been experiencing any of the above symptoms.

Scenario

A 35-year-old man is newly admitted to the ward. A random urine drug screen is positive for amphetamines and cannabis.

Take a history to assess for substance misuse.

Suggested approach

1. Good communication
2. Assess broadly for use of multiple substances, including onset, frequency, duration and method of use of each drug
3. Assess impact on functioning
4. Assess for comorbidity
5. Risk assessment

1. Good communication – Introduce and establish rapport, listen to the patient and empathize.

2. Assess broadly for use of multiple substances – Find out exactly which substances have been used and which are used regularly. The patient is unlikely to admit to every single drug so you should name substances and ask if the patient has tried them. Name several commonly used drugs including marijuana, cocaine, LSD, ecstasy, amphetamines and heroin. Assess onset, frequency and method of use of each drug. Elicit the quantities of each substance used, asking the patient to describe a typical day or week. Ask about pleasurable effects obtained and negative effects. Find out the duration of use and periods of abstinence. Ask how the patient copes with withdrawal symptoms. Ask about the route of use and whether the patient has been sharing needles. Ask whether the patient has contracted any diseases if he has been sharing needles. Ask if there is increased tolerance to the drugs and if more are being used. Ask if there is a compulsion to use drugs. Ask if there is a stereotyped pattern of usage.

3. Assess impact on functioning – How has drug use affected the patient in terms of his relationships, social and financial aspects of his life. Has it affected his self-care or other activities of daily living.

4. Assess for comorbidity – Enquire about comorbid depression, anxiety, personality or memory changes, or psychotic symptoms.

5. Risk assessment – Ask if the patient has got into any dangerous situations as a result of his drug taking. Ask if the patient has been involved in any criminal activity to fund his habit. Ask whether the patient has ever injected drugs and if so, is he aware of the danger of developing HIV or other blood-borne infections such as hepatitis from sharing needles?

Defining common conditions

- **Severe mental illness (SMI):** refers to the presence of a severe psychiatric disorder (eg schizophrenia, schizoaffective disorder, severe depression or bipolar disorder) accompanied by significant functional impairment, disruption of normal life tasks, periods of hospitalization and need for psychotropic medication.

- **Mental disorder:** the existence of a clinically recognizable set of symptoms or behaviour associated in most cases with distress and with interference with personal functions.

- **Personality disorder:** deeply ingrained and enduring behaviour patterns, manifesting themselves as inflexible responses to a broad range of personal and social situations.

Defining common conditions (cont.)

- **Schizophrenia:** a disorder characterized by distortions of thinking and perception and inappropriate or blunted affect. Hallucinations, delusions and thought disorder are common.

- **Hypomania:** persistent mild elevation of mood (for at least several days on end), increased energy and activity, and usually marked feelings of well-being and both physical and mental efficiency.

- **Mania:** elevated mood and psychomotor overactivity for at least 1 week duration.

- **Depression:** individual suffers low mood, low energy and anhedonia of at least 2 weeks duration.

- **PTSD:** a response to an exceptionally threatening event with typical repeated reliving of the trauma associated with numbness, detachment, avoidance and hyperarousal.

Defining common conditions

- **Dementia:** a syndrome resulting from disease of the brain, usually of a chronic or progressive nature, in which there is disturbance of multiple higher cortical functions, including memory, thinking, learning capacity and judgement.

- **Anorexia nervosa:** a disorder characterized by deliberate weight loss, induced and/or sustained by the patient.

- **Bulimia nervosa:** a syndrome characterized by repeated bouts of overeating and an excessive preoccupation with the control of body weight, leading the patient to adopt extreme measures so as to mitigate the 'fattening' effects of ingested food.

Defining common conditions (cont.)

- **Dependence syndrome (drugs or alcohol):** a cluster of physiological, behavioural and cognitive phenomena in which use of a substance or a class of substances takes on a much higher priority for a given individual than other behaviours that once had greater value.

- **Organic delusional (schizophrenia-like) disorder:** a disorder in which persistent or recurrent delusions dominate the clinical picture. The delusions may be accompanied by hallucinations but are not confined to their content. The general criteria for an organic disorder must be met.

Postnatal depression – Scottish Intercollegiate Guidelines (SIGN)

- Postnatal depression (PND) is regarded as any non-psychotic depressive illness of mild to moderate severity occurring during the first postnatal year.
- All women should be screened routinely for a history of depression or psychosis in previous pregnancies.
- All women should be screened for a history of depression in the current pregnancy. Note that emotional changes may mask a depression.
- If high risk give interpersonal therapy when pregnant, offer postnatal visits/antenatal preparation.
- If Edinburgh postnatal depression score is greater than 10 is suggested as a cut off for whole population screening.

Postnatal depression – Scottish Intercollegiate Guidelines (SIGN) (cont.)

- Note: The Edinburgh Postnatal Depression Scale is not diagnostic.
- When prescribing use the lowest effective dose (see Card 62).
- Do not routinely stop tricyclic antidepressants or SSRIs in early pregnancy. Risks of stopping medication should be carefully assessed in relation to the mother's history and potential risks.
- Psychosocial interventions should be considered when choosing treatment options for a mother diagnosed as suffering from PND.
- A multiprofessional assessment should be performed to determine if mother and baby should be admitted to a specialist unit.

NICE guidelines for self-harm

- **Assessment should consist of:**

  (i) Capacity to consent for further assessment (including assessment of presence of mental illness).

  (ii) Agitation.

  (iii) Previous history of self-harm.

  (iv) Presence of cognitions associated with suicide – depression/hopelessness/suicidal ideation.

- All assessments should be communicated to the GP and relevant mental health team. If thought to be at high risk of self-harm the patient should be offered intensive community outreach for at least 3 months consisting of supportive therapy, home treatment and a 24-hour contact should be made available. Alternatively refer for Dialectic Behaviour Therapy (DBT) if borderline personality disorder is thought to be associated with the self-harming behaviour.

Young people and deliberate self-harm

- Consider Gillick competence in children (if they are under 16 but have capacity they may be able to make a decision to accept treatment even if the parents disagree).
- If admission is needed admit to paediatric and not to the psychiatric ward.
- Advise parents to remove all medications and other means of self-harm at home.
- If there is a history of recurrent self-harm, offer developmental group psychotherapy.
- Assessment should consist of: child protection issues, collateral history from social services, family and school.

Older patients and deliberate self-harm

- Any DSH in a person over 65 should be considered attempted suicide until proven otherwise.
- Pay attention to presence of cognitive impairment, physical ill health, social and home situation.

Bipolar affective disorder

Bipolar affective disorder – NICE guidelines

Assessment, recognition, diagnosis

Primary care – Urgent referral for patients with mania or severe depression at risk to self or others

Referral for patients with history of overactive, disinhibited behaviour > 4 days ± depression

Secondary care – Assess symptoms, past history, triggers, social and personal functionality, stressors

Consider substance misuse and differentiate comorbiding eg psychosis/personality disorder

Risk assessment on first diagnosis, form a crisis plan considering early warning signs.

Mania/Hypomania

Stop antidepressant

If on antimania previously, if on an antipsychotic check dose and decrease if necessary

If response is inadequate, consider adding lithium or valproate

If on lithium check levels and ensure optimal dose is given

If on valproate increase dose until side effects limit further increase/until symptoms improve

In severe mania, if on lithium/valproate, consider adding an antipsychotic and gradually increasing dose of the original drug.

Maudsley algorithm for treatment of rapid cycling bipolar affective disorder

- Withdraw antidepressant →
- Optimize mood stabilizer →
- Combine two mood stabilizers →
- Add olanzapine/clozapine/nimodopine (Ca$^+$ channel blocker)/thyroxine/lamotrigine.

Post-traumatic stress disorder (PTSD)

NICE guidelines

- NB for a diagnosis the event leading to the PTSD has to be life threatening. Screening for PTSD in survivors of disasters is a useful measure. Debriefing may have a negative effect on prognosis and should not be offered.
- **General principles:** Treat any co-morbid axis 1 diagnosis (eg substance misuse/depression). Support the family. Consider cultural sensitivities pertinent to the situation.
- **Treatment:** (i) Watchful waiting. (ii) Trauma focused CBT/eye movement desensitization therapy (EMDR). (iii) Short term hypnotic. (iv) If no improvement with psychological therapies try: paroxetine or mirtazepine; amitryptiline or phenelzine; olanzapine as a final adjunct. Continue any medication for at least 12 months after recovery. (v) Do not offer other forms of psychotherapy or alternative therapies such as relaxation therapy as it avoids dealing with the traumatic event. (vi) If at high risk of suicide review weekly, otherwise review 2–4 weekly. (vii) In children with PTSD use psychological therapies. Medications are not recommended.

NICE guidelines for depression

Steps 1–2: Watchful waiting/self-help – mild depression

- Computer CBT.
- Activity scheduling.
- Exercise programmes.

Step 3: Level of GP/CMHT interface – moderate–severe depression

- Give medication.
- Fluoxetine/citalopram are the best choice of SSRIs.
- Continue treatment for 6 months.
- NICE guidelines do not recommend St Johns Wort.

Step 4: Level of secondary care – treatment-resistant depression/atypical/psychotic depression

Here treatment should be attempted along the following steps:
1. First antidepressant (AD).
2. AD and cognitive behavioural therapy (CBT).
3. AD and CBT and lithium.
4. If two ADs have failed start venlafaxine.
5. Augmentation, ie SSRI and mirtazapine.
6. Phenelzine (particularly indicated for atypical depression).
7. Refer to tertiary services.

Step 5: ECT

● Inpatient treatment and crisis response are the only level at which ECT is indicated. ECT is no longer recommended for maintenance treatment.

Other recommendations

● **Do not use**
carbamazepine/lamotrigine/pindolol/buspirone/valproate/thyroxine/benzodiazepines. Keep on maintenance treatment for 2 years if two or more episodes have occurred. If on combination antidepressant treatment, keep patient on both medications for at least 6 months then withdraw adjunct first.

NICE guidelines for schizophrenia (card 1 of 2)

Acute episode

1. Atypical antipsychotic treatment should be first line.
2. No loading doses. Use lowest possible dose.
3. If on typical and relapsed change to atypical.
4. Don't give two antipsychotics at the same time apart from short change over periods.
5. If no response change class of drugs.
6. When recovered let patient write their account in the notes.
7. On recovery full package of family therapy (FT), cognitive behavioural therapy (CBT) and occupational therapy (OT) should be offered.
8. Continue drugs for 1–2 years once well.
9. Gradual withdrawal after this. Monitor drug free for further 1–2 years.

Relapse prevention

● Continue medication and FT/CBT/OT as above. Monitor side-effects closely which NICE defines as:
  —Akathasia/EPSE
  —Weight gain/diabetes
  —Sexual dysfunction/hyperprolactinaemia
  —Oversedation
  —Eye signs.

Rapid tranquilization

● Use minimum dose possible.

● Never seclude if intoxicated on alcohol or drugs.

● If IM typical antipsychotic is given, give an IM anticholinergic as well.

● Make steps afterwards to re-establish the therapeutic relationship with the patient.

NICE guidelines for schizophrenia (card 2 of 2)

Treatment resistance

1. Check compliance

2. Exclude substance misuse

3. Exclude physical illness

4. Re-confirm diagnosis

5. Consider psychological therapies

6. Try risperidone or olanzapine if not tried already

7. In cases refractory to 2 other antipsychotics at optimal doses given for an adequate trial period, consider clozapine.

Clozapine augmentation – Maudsley guidelines

● Additional medication to consider adding in cases refractory to clozapine treatment include:
  —Sulpiride
  —Lamotrigine
  —Risperidone
  —EPA fish oil
  —Haloperidol
  —ECT.

Pathways to care

● If less than 35 years old and within first 3 years of illness, or new to services, patients should be referred to an early intervention service or to a crisis response/assertive outreach team with an aim to treat out of hospital.

Obsessive-compulsive disorder – NICE guidelines

General principles

- For patients with mild functional impairment first offer psychological therapies – Exposure and Response Prevention (ERP) up to 10 hours per patient or offer SSRI if unable to engage in ERP.

- For patients with moderate functional impairment, offer a choice of an SSRI or more intensive cognitive behavioural therapy (with ERP) – more than 10 hours per patient.

- Provide adequate information and support, liase with primary care, encourage family involvement if appropriate.

Obsessive-compulsive disorder – **NICE** guidelines (cont.)

Stepped care approach

Step 1 – Level of individuals/public organizations/NHS. Increase awareness and knowledge about OCD and where to seek help if necessary

Steps 2 and 3 – Primary care, practice nurses, primary care mental health workers. Recognition and assessment/initial treatment – discussion of treatment options, involve family and carers. May offer brief individual or group CBT (ERP) or an SSRI or both.

Step 4 – Level of secondary care. OCD with comorbidity or poor response to initial treatment – CBT (ERP), SSRI, alternative SSRI, clomipramine or combined treatments.

Step 5 – Specialist OCD service. OCD with significant comorbidity or severe functional impairment – SSRI or clomipramine or CBT (ERP) or combination of both SSRI/clomipramine and CBT (ERP).

Step 6 – Inpatient care/intensive treatment programmes. OCD associated with risk to life/severe self-neglect or severe distress/disability. Treatment as in step 5 or consider augmenting SSRI/clomipramine with an alternative medication.

Anorexia nervosa – physical management

Managing weight gain

- Aim for average weekly weight gain of 0.5–1 kg in inpatient settings and 0.5 kg in outpatient settings. This requires about 3500–7000 calories a week.
- Provide regular physical monitoring and consider multivitamin/multimineral supplement for both inpatients and outpatients.
- Total parenteral nutrition should be reserved only for significant gastrointestinal dysfunction.

Managing risk

- Inform patients and carers about potential physical risks.
- Involve physicians appropriately.
- Oestrogen administration only in adults if bone density problems exist.

Anorexia nervosa – inpatient care

- For patients with moderate or high physical risk/not improving with outpatient treatment/who have significant risk of suicide or severe self-harm.
- Admit to setting that can provide skilled services of refeeding with careful physical monitoring and in combination with psychosocial interventions.
- Psychological therapies with focus on symptoms and weight gain should be undertaken. Focus should be on eating behaviour and attitudes to weight and shape. Rigid behaviour modification programmes should not be used. Psychological input should continue for 12 months post discharge. Types of therapies can include: cognitive analytic therapy (CAT); cognitive behaviour therapy (CBT); interpersonal therapy (IPT); focal psychodynamic psychotherapy; family interventions focusing explicitly on eating disorders.
- Feeding against the will of the patient should be a last resort and only under Mental Health Act 1983 or Children Act 1989.

Anorexia nervosa – outpatient care

- Psychological therapies for 6 months minimum as above.
- Medications should be used with caution as depression and other comorbidity may improve with weight gain alone.
- Avoid using drugs which cause QTc prolongation. ECG monitoring should be undertaken if drugs are used which could affect cardiac function.

Bulimia nervosa

- First step – consider an evidence based self-help programme.
- Psychological treatment should be the key form of treatment.
- For adults – cognitive behaviour therapy (CBT) for 16–20 sessions over 4–5 months.
- If no response to CBT, try Interpersonal Therapy (IPT).
- Consider trial of an antidepressant drug as an alternative or in combination with a self-help programme.

Bulimia nervosa (cont.)

- SSRIs are the first choice as they are the most tolerable in terms of side-effects.
- Effective dose of fluoxetine is higher than in depression at 60 mg daily.
- Careful monitoring of physical risks should be undertaken including assessment of fluid and electrolyte balance where vomiting is frequent or there is frequent use of laxatives.

Answer True or False

Carbamazepine is a potent enzyme inducer.

True

Potent enzyme inducers include

- Carbamazepine.
- Phenytoin.
- Phenobarbital.

Enzyme inhibitors include

- Cimetidine.
- Diltiazem.
- Sodium valproate.
- Isoniazid.
- Metronidazole.
- Verapamil.
- Allopurinol.
- Chloramphenicol.
- Imipramine.
- Sulphonamides.
- Phenothiazines.

Answer True or False

1. The plenum temporale is situated on the anterior part of inferior temporal lobe.

2. Alexia without agraphia occurs in anterior cerebral artery lesions.

1 False – The plenum temporale encompasses the Wernicke's area and is located on the dorsal surface of the temporal lobe. This region is thought to be implicated in schizophrenia.

2 False – Anterior cerebral artery lesions – (i) upper motor neurone (UMN) palsy of foot and lower limb on contralateral side; (ii) sensory loss on contralateral side – foot and lower limb; (iii) urinary problems. **Posterior cerebral artery lesions** – (i) alexia without agraphia in left posterior cerebral artery lesions; (ii) Weber's syndrome; (iii) UMN palsy of whole contralateral side; (iv) ipsilateral oculomotor nerve palsy; (v) superior homonymous quadrantinopia.

Answer True or False

1. **HIV enters the** brain via infected macrophages.

2. Seizures are seen in tuberous sclerosis.

1 True – HIV-1 is a haematogenously spread virus that most likely gains entry into the brain within blood-derived macrophages.

2 True – Tuberous sclerosis is a rare multisystem genetic disease which causes benign tumours to grow in the brain and other organs including kidneys, eyes, lungs and skin. It commonly affects the central nervous system leading to seizures, developmental delay, behavioural problems, skin abnormalities and kidney disease.

Answer True or False

Astasia abasia may be a feature of dissociative disorders.

True

Astasia abasia is the inability to stand or walk in the absence of neurological abnormalities and may occur in functional dissociative psychiatric illnesses. Dissociative disorders:

Dissociative amnesia
Inability to recall information, usually about stressful or traumatic events in a person's life. Often abrupt onset after trauma. Patients are usually alert before and after the amnesia occurs. A few patients report slight clouding of consciousness during the period immediately before and after the amnesia onset. Preexisting depression and anxiety are common features in the history. Amnesia may be localized – few hours to few days; generalized – loss of memory for whole life or selective for certain events. Usually recovers spontaneously.

Dissociative fugue
Unusual and dramatic behaviour – patients travel far away from their home or work in a purposeful way for days at a time. They may take on an entirely or partially new identity and have amnesia for their past. They fail to remember important aspects of their previous identity (name, family, work). Persons with a history of alcoholism, personality disorder or other psychiatric illness are predisposed although the condition appears largely physiological in origin.

Dissociative identity disorder
See card 31 for more details.

Depersonalization disorder
See card 31 for more details.

Answer True or False

1. Delusional disorder usually precedes dementia.

2. Normal pressure hydrocephalus causing dementia is potentially reversible.

3. Personality changes before memory changes suggest Pick's disease rather than Alzheimer's disease.

4. Having a seizure is more suggestive of Pick's disease than Alzheimer's disease.

1 False

2 True – Abnormal gait, urinary incontinence and dementia are reversible when the condition is treated.

3. True – The first symptoms of Pick's disease are often personality change and a decline in function at work and at home.

4. False

Answer True or False

According to Donald Winnicott, a transitional object is considered the same as a 'good enough mother'.

False

- **A transitional object** is an item such as a blanket or teddy bear that enables a child to move away from an attachment figure and explore the world around them. It is seen as a method of providing security. It is described as transitional because it is thought to lie in the child's mind between their unconscious 'phantasy' of the idealized mother and the real world in which the mother is not so perfect. It is the child's way of adapting to loss of the phantasy of the idealized mother.

- **The 'good enough mother'** was described by Winnicott and describes the interaction between mother and baby in the weeks and months after childbirth. The mother supplies an environment in which the infant is contained and experiences life. The mother does not need to be perfect but needs to be a 'good enough mother' – for bonding to take place adequately and to ensure that the child forms a secure attachment and develops in good health. The infant learns to tolerate the frustration of learning that the mother will not always be present and this is seen as part of healthy development. Winnicott described a 'primary maternal preoccupation' in which the mother's attention is directed to her child in early infancy and thus forms a couple bond.

Answer True or False

1. A lesion in Broca's area results in an expressive aphasia.

2. The limbic system has been implicated in neuropathological studies of schizophrenia.

1 True – A lesion in Broca's area in the frontal lobe results in an expressive aphasia. Comprehension of speech is intact. A lesion in Wernicke's area results in a receptive aphasia with fluent speech. Comprehension of others speech is poor.

2 True – Functional neuroimaging has shown decreased activation of the frontal lobes in people with schizophrenia particularly when required to perform a task. There is also a decreased density of neuropil and the intertwined axons and dendrites of neurones in the frontal lobes. The limbic system includes the hippocampus, the fornix, the mamillary bodies, the anterior nucleus of the thalamus and the cingulate gyrus. It also includes the amygdala, septum, basal forebrain, nucleus accumbens and orbitofrontal cortex.

Answer True or False

Personality change is a late feature of Huntington's disease.

False

Huntington's disease characteristics

- A genetic disease transmitted in an autosomal dominant fashion with 100% penetrance; hence 50% of offspring are affected. The disease is characterized by a combination of progressive dementia and worsening chorea.

Aetiology

- Genetic defect in trinucleotide repeat of CAG on chromosome 4.

Characteristics

- Usually age of onset is in third and fourth decades of life. Deteriorating condition over 10–12 years to death.
- ***Changes in personality or mood may be the earliest signs of the disease.***
- Psychomotor slowing.
- Difficulty performing complex tasks.
- Characterized by: (i) dementia; (i) chorea (characterized by tics, jerks and involuntary movements, grimacing and dysarthria); (iii) autosomal dominant inheritance (family history).
- Depression, anxiety and psychosis are common features (60–80% of patients) even from the early stages of the illness.
- Memory, language and insight are relatively intact until the late stage of the disease when full dementia sets in.
- EEG shows diffuse slowing. PET shows decreased metabolism in the basal ganglia. MRI reveals basal ganglia atrophy as well as dilation of ventricles and atrophy of the head of the caudate
- Haloperidol may reduce movement disorder.

Answer True or False

Amphetamines act by enhancing cholinergic transmission.

False

- **Amphetamines are involved in the dopaminergic system and cause an increased release of dopamine** from the nucleus accumbens. This nucleus receives afferents from dopaminergic cells located in the ventral tegmental area and it is a convergence site for stimuli coming from the amygdala, hippocampus, entorrhinal area, anterior cingulate area and part of the temporal lobe (the so-called limbic system). It also has efferent projections for the septus, hypothalamus, anterior cingulate area and the frontal lobes. Due to its afferent and efferent connections the nucleus accumbens plays an important role in the regulation of emotion, motivation and cognition.

- **Mechanism of action of other drugs – Alcohol:** modulates GABA function, agonist at GABAa receptors. Also acts as an NMDA antagonist and causes decreased release of calcium ions. Modulation of NMDA may lead to memory changes associated with long term use. May also be associated with low or high 5HT levels leading to mood/behaviour changes (low 5HT associated with impulsivity, high 5HT associated with anxiety). **Acamprosate**: antagonizes the excitatory effects of NMDA (glutamate) in the brain and stimulates inhibitory GABA-ergic transmission. **Disulfiram:** inhibits aldehyde dehydrogenase. **Naltrexone:** non-selective opioid receptor antagonist. **Opioids (heroin, methadone, codeine):** act as agonists at μ (analgesia, positive reinforcement, euphoria) and κ receptors (dysphoria, sedation). **PCP and ketamine:** NMDA antagonists. **LSD:** 5HT2a agonist. **Marijuana:** tetrahydrocannabinol alters cerebellar and hippocampal neuronal activity.

Answer True or False

Perinatal complications are a risk factor for bipolar affective disorder.

False

● There may be an association between perinatal complications and BPAD but such a link has not yet been clearly established.

● **Risk factors for BPAD:**

   ● M=F (not more common in either sex).

   ● History of cyclothymia.

   ● FHx of BPAD (25% risk if one parent has the disorder, 50-75% chance if both parents affected).

   ● FHx of unipolar depression.

   ● Genetic factors – 43% monozygotic twin concordance, 6% for dizygotic twins.

Answer True or False

1. Maternity blues are present in 50% of new mothers.

2. The Edinburgh Postnatal Depression Scale is self-completed.

1 True - Maternity blues is the term given to a mild and transient disturbance in mood which occurs between the third and sixth day after delivery. Common features include crying, fatigue, anxiety, irritability, feelings of helplessness and lability of mood. Symptoms last from a few hours to a few days. Estimates of incidence vary between 50% and 70%, and it is commonest in women having their first baby.

2 True – The Edinburgh Postnatal Depression Scale was designed to assist primary care professionals to detect postnatal depression. It is a self-rated questionnaire filled out by the mother. Postnatal depression usually occurs from 1 week after delivery and may last for several months. It occurs in about 10% of women after delivery. It is more common in women with a personal or family history of depression.

Answer True or False

Amenorrhea is a recognized complication of bulimia nervosa.

True – Amenorrhoea commonly occurs in anorexia and may occur in bulimia nervosa also.

Complications of eating disorders associated with weight loss

- **Cardiac** – cardiac arrhythmias including atrial and ventricular tachycardia, prolonged QT interval, bradycardia and sudden death.
- **Cachexia** – loss of fat, muscle mass, reduced thyroid metabolism (low T3 syndrome), cold intolerance and difficulty maintaining core body temperature.
- **Dermatological** – lanugo (fine baby-like hair over body), oedema.
- **GI** – delayed gastric emptying, bloating, constipation, abdominal pain.
- **Haematological** – leucopenia
- **Neuropsychiatric** – abnormal taste sensation, mild cognitive disorder, apathetic depression.
- **Reproductive** – amenorrhoea, low LH and FSH.
- **Skeletal** – osteoporosis.

Complications of eating disorders associated with vomiting

- **Dental** – erosion of dental enamel leading to tooth decay.
- **GI** – salivary gland and pancreatic inflammation and enlargement with increase in serum amylase, oesophageal and gastric erosion
- **Metabolic** – electrolyte abnormalities, particularly hypokalaemic hypochloraemic alkalosis, hypomagnesaemia.
- **Neuropsychiatric** – seizures, mild neuropathies, fatigue and weakness.

Answer True or False

1. **Anorexia** is commonly associated with overeating.

2. **Pickwickian syndrome** is associated with overeating.

3. **Klein–Levin syndrome** is associated with overeating.

1 False – **Anorexia nervosa** can be divided into two types: binge type or restrictive. The binge type is relatively uncommon.

2 True – **Pickwickian syndrome** is a complex of symptoms that primarily affects patients with extreme obesity (100% overweight). Main effects are on the respiratory system with excessive daytime sleepiness, shortness of breath and facial flushing.

3 True – **Klein–Levin syndrome** is a rare condition characterized by periodic episodes of hypersomnia (each lasting for one or several weeks) intervened by periods of normal sleep. It first appears in adolescence, usually in boys, and is accompanied by bulimia, apathy, irritability, confusion, depression, disorientation and memory impairment during wakeful periods. It is not classified as either an eating disorder or a sleep disorder. It is considered likely to be a neurological syndrome and is believed to reflect a frontal lobe or hypothalamic disturbance. The syndrome is self-limited and remission occurs in most cases by age 40.

Answer True or False

1. **Delusional** perception can be secondary to hallucinations.

2. **Pseudocyesis and Couvade** syndrome are interchangeable.

1 False - **Delusional perception** is a primary delusion and therefore cannot be secondary to hallucinations. A primary delusion is one which arises out of the blue. There are four types of primary delusion – mood, perception, intuition and atmosphere.

2 False – **Pseudocyesis** is an imaginary pregnancy in a woman. It usually results from a strong desire for motherhood. In the absence of conception, the menstrual periods stop, the abdomen becomes enlarged and the breasts swell and even secrete milk, mimicking a genuine pregnancy. The uterus and cervix may show signs of pregnancy, urine tests may be falsely positive, and the woman may report sensations of fetal movements.

Couvade syndrome is a sympathetic pregnancy in a man. The aetiology is unknown and it usually resolves spontaneously.

Answer True or False

A WAIS with a 15-point difference between verbal and performance suggests an organic brain lesion.

True

- A 15-point difference between the two categories does suggest an organic brain lesion.

- The WAIS is the most standardized and widely used intelligence test in current clinical practice. David Weschler invented intelligence tests. He designed three tests:
  —WPPSI-R for preschool (primary school) children 3–7 years
  —WISC III-R for children 6–16 years
  —WAIS-III (Weschler Adult Intelligence Scale).

- The WAIS-III for ages 16 years and above consists of two areas:
  —**Verbal set:** divided into six areas tested (digit span, vocabulary, maths, etc.)
  —**Performance set:** 11 areas (picture completion, block design, etc.).

Answer True or False

In psychodynamic theory, Freud's dream work stages include secondary elaboration.

True

Freud's dream work stages are based on his paper 'The Interpretation of Dreams'. Freud believed dreams have a symbolic nature and are the gateway to our unconscious. The stages are:

1. **Condensation:** two or more latent (hidden) thoughts are combined to make one 'manifest' dream image or situation.

2. **Displacement:** emotions or desires towards something or someone are directed towards a meaningless unrelated object in the manifest dream.

3. **Symbolization:** complex or vague concepts are then converted into a dream image, Freud believed this was to do with sexual desires.

4. **Secondary elaboration:** the dream is actually made to make sense (takes on a full form) by having some relevance to the person's everyday life.

Answer True or False

A WAIS score of greater than 125 is found in 10% of the population.

False

A WAIS score of greater than 125 is found in 5% of the population. The lowest 2.5% have an IQ below 70 (mental retardation) and approximately 2% of the population have an IQ above 130.

Answer True or False

Phenytoin can cause alopecia.

False

Side-effects of phenytoin include:

- **CNS** – Drowsiness, ataxia, memory problems, dysarthria, confusion, tremor
- **GI** – Gingival hyperplasia, diarrhoea, constipation, nausea, vomiting, liver damage.
- **Haematological** – Agranulocytosis, aplastic anaemia, haemolytic anaemia, leucocytosis, monocytosis, anaemia.
- **Dermatological** – Measles-like rash, scarlatiniform, maculopapular and urticarial rashes. Rarely: drug-induced lupus, Stevens–Johnson syndrome and toxic epidermal necrolysis.
- **Ophthalmic** – Diplopia, nystagmus, conjunctivitis.

Answer True or False

Psychomotor retardation is generally considered to be a negative symptom of schizophrenia.

True

Positive and negative symptoms of schizophrenia (Andreasen *et al.* 1983)

- Positive symptoms include hallucinations, delusions, formal thought disorder and bizarre behaviour.
- Negative symptoms include – **mnemonic: 7 As – A**ffective blunting, **A**logia (impoverished thinking and speech), **A**volition, **A**pathy, **A**nhedonia, **A**sociality, **A**ttention disturbance.

Liddle's classification (confirmed by a PET study of regional cerebral blood flow)

- Psychomotor poverty syndrome: there is poverty of speech, flattened affect and decreased spontaneous movement.
- Disorganization syndrome: disorders of thought form and inappropriate affect.
- Reality distortion syndrome: there are delusions and hallucinations.

Answer True or False

Asyndesis refers to a disorder in which thoughts do not join together to form one coherent concept.

True

- **Asyndesis** – There is lack of connection between one thought and another.
- Other types of thought disorder:

  —**Metonym** – An inappropriate or imprecise but related word is used in place of the correct word in a sentence.

  —**Neologism** – A new word that has no meaning is created.

  —**Echolalia** – Automatic and pointless repetition of another person's words or phrases.

  —**Verbigeration** – Imitation of another person's phrases in a stereotyped manner.

  —**Palilalia** – Repetition of a word from an individual's own spoken words.

  —**Logoclonia** – Repetition of words or phrases, particularly the end syllables.

  —**Logorrhoea:** excessive flow of words or pressure of speech as occurs in mania.

Answer True or False

1. **Anankastic personality disorder is associated with magical undoing.**

2. **Paranoid schizoid position can lead to psychological difficulties.**

1 False – OCD is characterized by three defence mechanisms: **mnemonic** – **URI** (see card 77) – Magical **U**ndoing, **R**eaction formation, **I**solation.

Not for anankastic personality disorder.

2 False – Paranoid schizoid position is a psychodynamic theory formulated by Melanie Klein. It has no relation to psychological difficulties. Exam candidates need to understand the difference between psychology and psychodynamic theory. The two are different schools and should not be put together in this way.

Answer True or False

1. St John's Wort enhances the effect of SSRIs.

2. Trazodone has a weak antagonistic effect on serotonin.

1 True St John's Wort is believed to act on serotonin and therefore has a similar mechanism of action to SSRIs. A serotonin syndrome has been known to occasionally occur when people take the two in combination.

2 False Trazodone is an example of a dual serotonin 2A and serotonin reuptake inhibitor. Its effects are: **powerful** antagonism of serotonin 2A receptors and less powerful blockade of serotonin reuptake. Nefazodone is a similar agent.

Answer True or False

Children under 1 year of age are scared of loud noises.

True

Most common fears – up to 1 year of age

- Loud noises.
- Fear of animals, insects.
- Separation from parents.
- Falling.

1–6 years of age

- Strangers.
- Animals.
- Darkness.
- Monsters.

6–11 years of age

- Separation anxiety.
- Death.

12–16 years of age

- Fears about social rejection, sexual anxieties.
- Worries about personal achievement.

Answer True or False

Dopamine is a precursor of noradrenaline.

True

- **Tyrosine** is hydroxylated → **DOPA** (dihydroxyphenylalanine) by action of tyrosine hydroxylase.
- **DOPA** is decarboxylated → **dopamine** by DOPA decarboxylase.
- **Dopamine** → **noradrenaline** (converted by the action of dopamine β-hydroxylase).
- **Dopamine** is also metabolized by **MAO** (mitochondrial monoamine oxidase) and by **COMT** (catechol-O-methyltransferase) to form the end product **HVA** (homovanillic acid).

Answer True or False

Selective abstraction is a cognitive distortion.

True

Cognitive distortions according to Beck's cognitive theory of depression

- **Arbitrary inference** – Drawing the worst possible conclusions about a given problem without adequate evidence.
- **Selective abstraction** – Focusing on the worst aspects of past experiences, ie only the worst events are remembered.
- **Overgeneralization** – Drawing negative general conclusions about personal worth from one example of something that went wrong.
- **Minimization** – Good performance is underestimated.
- **Magnification** – Errors are overestimated.
- **Personalization** – A tendency to attribute all wrong doings to negatively perceived personal attributes.
- **Dichotomous thinking** – Black and white thinking such as 'all women think I'm ugly'.

Answer True or False

Perception of time is always altered in depersonalization

False

- Perception of time may be altered in depersonalization. There may be an alteration in the sense of duration or perspective of time. This is not always the case however.

- Depersonalization is a term used to describe a change in the awareness of the self in which the individual feels as if he/she is unreal. This **feeling** must be differentiated from an **experience** of unreality as is often seen in psychotic patients.

- **Aspects of depersonalization** – May occur in healthy individuals. There is often a comorbid mood or neurotic disorder. Usually experiences are ego dystonic. Often felt to be subjectively unpleasant. Emotional numbing. Changes in body experience. Changes in sensory perception: visual/auditory/tactile/gustatory/olfactory. Loss of feelings of agency. Distortions in experience of time. Changes in subjective experience of memory. Heightened self-observation. Feelings of thoughts being empty. Subjective feeling of inability to evoke images.

Answer True or False

Neurofibrillary tangles are found as often in Pick's disease as in Alzheimer's dementia.

False

Pick's disease versus Alzheimer's dementia

- Pick's disease is more common in women than in men, and especially if there is a first degree relative with the condition.

- Similar to Alzheimer's disease in some respects although Pick's disease is more often characterized by personality and behavioural changes (disinhibition, aggression, rudeness towards others) in the early stages with relative preservation of other cognitive functions.

- Pick's disease is characterized by atrophy in the frontotemporal regions with neuronal loss, gliosis and neuronal Pick bodies (these are not always seen in post-mortem and are not necessary for the diagnosis). Pick bodies are different from the neurofibrillary tangles seen in Alzheimer's disease. **Neurofibrillory tangles are much less common in Pick's disease.**

- Features of Kluver–Bucy syndrome (hypersexuality, hyperorality, placidity) are more common in Pick's disease than in Alzheimer's. Agnosia and apraxia may occur in Pick's disease but are much less common than in Alzheimer's dementia and usually occur later in the course of the disease.

Answer True or False

1. DSM IV is hierarchical.

2. DSM IV includes psychosocial stressors on Axis III.

3. DSM IV uses a dimensional rather than a categorical classification.

4. DSM IV uses operational criteria.

1 False   2 False   3 True   4 True

The DSM uses a multiaxial or multidimensional approach to diagnosing on the basis that it is rare that other factors in a person's life do not impact on their mental health. It uses operational criteria and assesses five dimensions:

- Axis I – Major mental disorders, developmental disorders and learning disabilities.
- Axis II – Underlying pervasive or personality conditions, as well as mental retardation.
- Axis III – Non-psychiatric medical condition(s).
- Axis IV – Social functioning and impact of symptoms.
- Axis V – Global Assessment of Functioning (on a scale from 0 to 100).

Answer True or False

Hyperresponsiveness of noradrenergic neurones in the locus coeruleus may be responsible for recurrent flashbacks in PTSD sufferers.

True

- **Risk factors in PTSD: predisposing psychological factors** – Hx of childhood trauma. Personality disorder: borderline, paranoid, antisocial or dependent. Lack of support. Recent excess alcohol intake. Female gender. F Hx of psychiatric illness. External perception of locus of control rather than internal.

- **Psychodynamic factors** – Reactivation of previously unresolved psychological conflict. Results in regression and use of defence mechanisms: repression, denial, reaction formation, magical undoing.

- **Cognitive factors** – Affected individuals unable to process and rationalize the trauma. Trauma (unconditioned stimulus) results in a fear response which is paired with a conditioned stimulus (reminders of the trauma, eg similar sounds, smells).

- **Biological factors:**
  - **Noradrenergic system** – strong evidence of altered function in the noradrenergic system in PTSD. 30–40% of PTSD patients report flashbacks after yohimbine administration.
  - **Opioid system** – Abnormality suggested by low beta endorphin concentrations.
  - **Corticotophin releasing factor (CRF) and the HPA Axis** – Blunted ACTH response to exogenous CRF. Suppression of cortisol enhanced by dexamethasone.

Answer True or False

Tourette's syndrome is more common in males than in females

True

- Tourette's syndrome
  - Three times more common in boys than in girls.
  - Occurs in 4–5 per 10,000 population.
  - Onset of the motor component usually occurs by 7 years of age.
  - Vocal tics emerge on average by 11 years.
  - Obsessive-compulsive disorder, attention problems and impulsivity have been associated with Tourette's.
- The disorder is characterized by multiple motor (usually beginning in face and neck and progressing downwards) and one or more vocal tics that occur many times a day and cause significant impairment in functioning.
- See card 16 for further details.

Answer True or False

Schizotypal disorder is in the same category as schizophrenia in the ICD10.

True

● Schizophrenia, schizotypal and delusional disorders is a category in ICD10 (F20–29).

● **Schizotypal disorder** – Characterized by eccentric behaviour and abnormalies of thinking and affect similar to those seen in schizophrenia. Any of the following may be present (ICD10):

—Inappropriate or constricted affect (individual appears cold and aloof)

—Behaviour or appearance that is odd, eccentric or peculiar

—Poor rapport with others and a tendency to social withdrawal

—Odd beliefs or magical thinking, influencing behaviour and inconsistent with social norms

—Suspiciousness or paranoid ideas

—Obsessive ruminations without inner resistance, often with dysmorphophobic, sexual or aggressive contents

—Unusual perceptual experiences including somatosensory or other illusions, depersonalization or derealization

—Vague, circumstantial, metaphorical, overelaborate or stereotyped thinking, manifested by odd speech or in other ways, without gross incoherence

—Occasional transient quasi-psychotic episodes with intense illusions, auditory or other hallucinations, and delusion-like ideas, usually occurring without external provocation Usually runs a chronic course. Occasionally may evolve into overt schizophrenia.

Answer True or False

1. **Social phobia** is more common in women than in men.

2. In **phobic anxiety** disorders, a good response to behaviour therapy is associated with **specific phobias**.

3. **Preparedness** occurs in simple phobias.

1 True – 60% female distribution (F:M = 3:2).

Sex distributions of some other neurotic disorders:

- Agoraphobia F:M = 4:1.
- Specific phobia F:M = 2:1.
- Panic disorder F:M = 2:1.
- Generalized anxiety disorder F:M = 2:1.
- Dissociative disorder F > M.
- Obsessive-compulsive disorder F:M = 1:1.
- Hypochondriasis F:M 1:1.

2 True – Good response is also associated with the degree of patient motivation as well as support from family and friends.

3 True – The preparedness theory of phobia holds that humans are biologically prepared to fear objects that threatened the survival of the species throughout its evolutionary history. This is thought to explain why children are scared of snakes from a very early age despite having no prior knowledge that they may be poisonous.

Answer True or False

1. Poor verbal fluency is an early feature of frontal lobe syndrome.

2. Confabulation is an essential feature of Wernicke–Korsakoff syndrome.

3. Confabulation in Wernicke–Korsakoff syndrome can include elements of true memory.

1 False – Poor verbal fluency tends to be a late feature of frontal lobe syndrome. Subtle personality changes tend to occur earlier on.

2 False – Confabulation is a common feature but is not essential for the diagnosis.

3 True – Confabulation may include elements of true memory. **Wernicke's encephalopaphy –** acute symptoms associated with chronic excess alcohol intake: Ataxia; ophthalmoplegia (ocular abnormalities in more than 80% of cases); nystagmus; confusion; vestibular dysfunction; anisocoria ; slow light reflex. Wernicke's encephalopathy is usually reversible with treatment with parenteral thiamine at high doses. It may either resolve or progress to Korsakoff's syndrome which is usually irreversible. **Korsakoff's syndrome** – chronic amnestic syndrome characterized by: impaired memory especially for recent events; anterograde amnesia in an alert and responsive person.

Answer True or False

1. **Repertory** grid is a specific test of intelligence.

2. Recency and primacy effects help recall in short term memory.

1 False – The repertory grid (Bannister) is not an intelligence test. George Kelly's personal construct theory emphasizes an individual's self-appraisal in studying his or her own personality. The theory is that a person's mental processes are psychologically channelled by the way they anticipate events. The repertory grid created by Bannister is a tool used between a patient and a therapist to consider the dimensions of the patient's personality – it is based on the personal construct theory.

2 True – **Primacy effect:** the tendency to remember the first few items on a list better than subsequent items. The first few items are most rehearsed and receive undivided attention and are therefore more likely to be stored in long term memory. **Recency effect:** the tendency to remember the last few items on a list. This is associated with storage of information in short term memory. For example, if asked to read a list of 15 items, there will be a tendency to remember the first and last few items on the list better than the middle items. This is because of the above effects. Primacy allows the first few items to be remembered better in the long term also. If there is a delay in recalling the items, the recency effect will be lost as items are only stored in short term memory.

Answer True or False

The risk of postpartum psychosis is 20% if there is one previous episode of postpartum psychosis.

Postpartum psychosis

- Incidence – 1–2 per 1000 births.
- 50–60% of cases are after birth of first child.

Risk factors

- 50% involve obstetric complications in labour.
- 50% of women affected have a family history of mood disorder.
- Personal or family history of schizophrenia or other psychotic illness.
- Past episode of postpartum psychosis – between 20% and 50% chance of recurrence in future pregnancy.

Answer True or False

1. Obsessive-compulsive disorder is more common in females than in males.

2. In obsessive-compulsive disorder there is increased glucose metabolism in the caudate nucleus.

1 False – Epidemiology

- Equal sex distribution (M = F).
- Most commonly occurs in early adulthood, mean age of onset is 20 years.
- Lifetime prevalence 2–3%.

2 True – Biological factors in OCD

- Serotonergic system – an abnormality in serotonin regulation has been identified as the disorder responds mainly to serotonergic drugs rather than drugs affecting other neurotransmitters.
- Brain imaging studies suggest altered function in neurocircuitry between the orbitofrontal cortex, caudate and thalamus. PET scans have shown increased glucose metabolism in the head of the caudate.
- Genetic factors – 35% of first-degree relatives are affected by this disorder.

Answer True or False

Patients suffering from Alzheimer's dementia are more likely to show deficits in verbal fluency than those suffering vascular dementia.

False

- **Vascular dementia cardinal features** – Difficulty sustaining attention. Executive dysfunction. Verbal fluency deficits. Onset may be sudden and presents with patchy cognitive deficits with a stepwise deterioration. Psychotic symptoms are uncommon.

- **Alzheimer's disease cardinal features – mnemonic: 5 A's** – **A**mnesia – memory problems – particularly recent, **A**phasia – speech deficits, language and comprehension problems, **A**praxia – problems performing tasks, **A**gnosia – difficulty recognizing familiar people or objects, **A**nomia – difficulty naming. Onset is usually slow and there is usually a slow decline in cognitive function. When insight is still present, depressive symptoms are common and psychotic symptoms are also common.

- **Risk factors for vascular dementia** – Alzheimer's disease, mild cognitive impairment, preexisting vascular disease, family history of dementia, Down's syndrome, head injury, increasing age.

Answer True or False

30% of depressed patients have elevated cortisol levels.

False

● About 50% have elevated cortisol levels.

Biological findings in depression

● **Serotonin** - Depletion of serotonin may precipitate depression.
● **Noradrenaline** - Correlation exists between downregulation of β-adrenergic receptors and antidepressant responses.

Neuroendocrine dysregulation

● Hypothalamic–pituitary–adrenal (HPA) axis dysfunction - About 50% of depressed patients have elevated cortisol levels and the cortisol levels are not suppressed normally by administration of dexamethasone.
● Thyroid disorders are found in 5–10% of depressed individuals. See card 46 for further details.
● Growth hormone - Depressed individuals have a blunted sleep-induced stimulation of growth hormone response although this has not been linked to sleep abnormalities in depression.

Answer True or False

Yalom described communalism as a curative factor in groups.

False

Yalom (1975) described 12 curative factors in groups which apply to group therapy – mnemonic: CAGED In Uniforms

C – Catharsis, Corrective recapitulation of the family group (2).
A – Altruism.
G – Group cohesiveness, Guidance (2).
E – Existential awareness.
D – Development of socializing techniques.
I – Insight, Interpersonal learning, Imitative behaviour (3).
U – Universality.

Rappaport's theory of the basic features of a therapeutic community – mnemonic: CPR Grade D

C – Communalism – equal treatment and shares for everyone.
P – Permissiveness – tolerance of disturbed behaviour.
R – Reality confrontation – regular feedback given to individuals on the results of their behaviour.
D – Democratization – abolition of hierarchy.

Answer True or False

1. **Depression** is more common in women than in men.

2. In those who have completed suicide, it has been found that there is an increased concentration of 5-HIAA in the CSF.

3. Failure of suppression of the Dexamethasone Suppression Test occurs in about 80% of people suffering from major depression.

1 True – Depression is more common in women. Completed suicide is more common in men.

2 False – It has been found that in depressed individuals there is decreased plasma tryptophan and decreased platelet 5HT uptake. There are low levels of CSF 5-hydroxyindole acetic acid (HIAA) in individuals who have completed suicide, although this is not a consistent finding.

3 False – Occurs in about 50–60% of depressed individuals but this is not specific to depression as failure of suppression in DST also occurs in other conditions including alcohol dependency and schizophrenia.

Options

A. Extracampine hallucination
B. Functional hallucination
C. Illusion
D. Synaesthesia
E. Pseudohallucination
F. Delusional perception
G. Autoscopy
H. Haptic hallucination
I. Synaesthesia
J. Hynagogic hallucination
K. Paranoid delusion
L. Hypnapompic hallucination
M. Reflex hallucination

Instructions

For each of the conditions described below, choose the most likely diagnosis from the list of options. Each option may be used once, more than once or not at all.

1. A 31-year-old man tells the ward doctor one day that his coffee tastes funny and says he believes this is because staff have been putting poison in it.
2. A 16-year-old boy on the medical ward is admitted following use of LSD. He says that when he sees the colour red he can also hear it, and the brighter the red, the louder the sound.
3. A patient tells you he hears a voice whispering to him in a female voice when he wakes up in the morning.

1. F. Delusional perception: a normal perception is given delusional meaning, eg a patient drinks coffee which looks very dark (normal perception). The coffee being dark is then given a delusional meaning, eg that the staff have been putting poison into it.

2. I. Synaesthesia: perception of one stimulus evokes a second stimulus sensation.

3. L. Hypnapompic hallucination: a vivid hallucination that occurs while waking up from sleep.

Options

A. Capgras' syndrome
B. Fregoli's syndrome
C. De Clarambault's syndrome
D. Couvade's syndrome
E. Cotard's syndrome

F. Pseudocyesis
G. Reduplicative paramnesia
H. Doppleganger
I. Folie à deux
J. Morbid jealousy

Instructions

For each of the conditions described below, choose the most likely diagnosis from the list of options. Each option may be used once, more than once or not at all.

1. A woman is referred to the outpatient clinic by her GP. Her menses stopped 2 months ago and she has developed abdominal distension and believes she is pregnant. She has had a home pregnancy test that was negative and she has seen an obstetrician who performed an ultrasound and this confirmed that she is not pregnant.
2. A 39-year-old man on the psychiatric ward says that one of the patients whom he does not know has been replaced by a friend of his.
3. A 47-year-old lady suffering schizophrenia says that she feels like she knows the street where the mental health unit is, and believes it is exactly the same as the street where she lives, even though she has never been there before.

1. F. Pseudocyesis: a false pregnancy. Often presents with many of the signs and symptoms of pregnancy and is similar to a real pregnancy in every way except for the presence of a foetus. Couvade's syndrome is a sympathetic pregnancy in a man.

2. B. Fregoli's syndrome: a delusional belief that a stranger has been replaced by someone familiar. Capgras' syndrome is the opposite – a belief that a stranger has replaced a familiar person.

3. G. Reduplicative paramnesia: a feeling that a familiar place has been duplicated.

Options

A. α_1	F. $5HT_{1a}$	K. Serotonin
B. α_2	G. $5HT_{2a}$	L. Noradrenaline
C. M_1	H. $5HT_{2c}$	M. H_1
D. M_5	I. $5HT_3$	N. Acetylcholine
E. GABA a	J. Glutamate	

Instructions

For each of the statements below, choose the most likely receptor(s) from the list of options. Each option may be used once, more than once or not at all.

1. Antipsychotics cause extrapyramidal side-effects as a result of dopamine receptor antagonism. Dopamine antagonism causes an increase in activity of which of the above receptors? (Choose one)
2. A patient on antipsychotics has developed weight gain, drowsiness and hypotension. Which of the above two receptors are responsible for these effects? (Choose two)
3. Valproic acid acts on which of the above receptors? (Choose two).
4. On which of the above receptors does mirtazapine act? (Choose five)

1. N: dopamine normally inhibits acetylcholine release. Dopamine antagonism therefore leads to an increase in acetylcholine activity which causes extrapyramidal symptoms.

2. A, M: α_1 blockade causes hypotension, dizziness and drowsiness. H_1 blockade causes weight gain.

3. E, J: valproic acid acts on calcium and sodium channels and enhances the inhibitory action of GABA as well as reducing the excitatory action of glutamate.

4. B, G, H, I, M: mirtazapine is a noradrenergic and serotonergic antidepressant. Its main mechanism of action is via alpha 2 blockade which leads to serotonin ($5HT_{1a}$) release. But it also blocks serotonin $5HT_{2a}$, $5HT_{2c}$, $5HT_3$ as well as H_1 receptors. Sedation and weight gain result from H_1 blockade.

Options

A. Amitriptyline
B. Imipramine
C. Citalopram
D. Amisulpiride
E. Donepezil
F. Venlafaxine
G. Lithium
H. Clozapine
I. Mirtazapine

Instructions

For each of the conditions described below, choose the most appropriate drug from the list of options. Each option may be used once, more than once or not at all.

1. A 31-year-old man was diagnosed with schizophrenia 4 years ago and initially his mental state improved whilst taking olanzapine orally. He has had three admissions over the last 4 years due to poor adherence to medication. He refuses to try depot medication and has now had another relapse of his illness. He tells you one of the reasons he stopped taking olanzapine was because it made him put on weight and he feels very conscious about this.
2. A 76-year-old man with a history of benign prostatic hypertrophy becomes depressed with symptoms of low mood, anhedonia, low energy as well as loss of appetite.
3. A 26-year-old lady has been experiencing depression for the last 6 months. She has tried an SSRI antidepressant but it has not helped improve her symptoms. She has been sleeping excessively.

1. D. Amisulpiride: is associated with a low risk of weight gain. Clozapine and olanzapine have a high risk of weight gain. Risperidone and quetiapine are associated with a moderate risk of weight gain.

2. C. Citalopram: an SSRI such as citalopram would be the best choice, as it does not have alpha 1 antagonism which can aggravate benign prostatic hypertrophy. Tricyclics cause alpha 1 antagonism and should therefore be avoided.

3. F. Venlafaxine: when an SSRI has failed, a different class of antidepressant such as venlafaxine should be tried first. Mirtazapine would not be the best choice in this case due to its sedating effects which would not help her given her excessive sleeping.

Options

A. Modelling
B. Operant conditioning
C. Classical conditioning
D. Positive reinforcement
E. Negative reinforcement
F. Stimulus generalization
G. Fixed ratio reinforcement
H. Variable ratio reinforcement
I. Shaping
J. Extinction

Instructions

For each of the scenarios described below, choose the most likely option from the list above. Each option may be used once, more than once or not at all.

1. An advertising company puts a picture of a beautiful woman leaning against a car that it wants to sell.
2. A dog comes down to the kitchen whenever he hears the owner come home and open and close the door at 6pm every day. The dog knows that the owner gives him his food when he gets in from work every day. Sometimes the dog hears a similar sound to the door being closed and rushes down to the kitchen.
3. An 11-year-old girl is asked to brush her teeth at night before going to sleep. She refuses to do this despite encouragement from her mother. Eventually her mother stops giving her encouragement and scolds her for not brushing her teeth. She continues not to brush her teeth. The mother then takes away her pocket money and the girl then starts brushing her teeth.

1. C. Classical conditioning: the advertising company is associating a beautiful lady with the car so that when an individual thinks of the car they will think of a beautiful lady.

2. F. Stimulus generalization: the dog has learnt to associate the sound of the closing door at 6pm with food. The dog hears similar sounds which he then also associates with the food.

3. B. Operant conditioning: punishment is used as a method of changing behaviour.

Options

A. General Health Questionnaire (GHQ)
B. Burden Questionnaire
C. Hachinski Ischemic Score
D. Alzheimer's Disease Quality of Life
Questionnaire
E. Mini Mental State Exam
F. Wisconsin Card Sorting Test
G. Benton Revised Visual Retention Test
H. Clinical Dementia Rating Scale

Instructions

Read the short short case history and for each of the following questions choose the most likely diagnosis from the list of options. Each option may be used once, more than once or not at all.

A woman has brought her 83-year-old father to the accident and emergency department saying she has been finding it difficult to look after him recently as he has become increasingly irritable and verbally aggressive toward her over the last few weeks:

1. Which scale could be used to assess the mood of the daughter?
2. Which test could be used to assess the global cognitive function of the patient?
3. If his global cognitive functions were found to be normal, which test could be used to specifically assess his frontal lobe functions?

363

1. A. General Health Questionnaire: a self-administered questionnaire which focuses on two major areas: (i) the inability to carry out normal functions and (ii) the appearance of new and distressing symptoms. The General Health Questionnaire (GHQ) is available in the following versions:

GHQ-60: full 60-item questionnaire.
GHQ-30: short form without questions on physical illness.
GHQ-28: a 28-item scaled version – assesses somatic symptoms, anxiety, insomnia, social dysfunction and depression.
GHQ-12: quick, reliable and sensitive short form – best for research.

2. E. Mini Mental State Exam (MMSE): consists of the following:

Orientation to Time (5 points) and Place (5), Registration (3), Concentration (5), Recall (3), Naming (2), Repetition (1), Three Stage Command (3), Write a sentence (1), Follow a task (eg close your eyes)(1), Draw intersecting pentagons (1). Total = 30 points.

3. F. Wisconsin Card Sorting Test: assesses frontal lobe functions. It primarily tests judgement, perseveration and abstract abilities.

Options

A. Cyclothymia
B. Depression
C. Dysthymia
D. Bipolar affective disorder
E. Mania
F. Hypomania
G. Rapid cycling bipolar affective disorder
H. Mixed anxiety and depressive disorder

Instructions

For each of the conditions described below, choose the most likely diagnosis from the list of options. Each option may be used once, more than once or not at all.

1. A 37-year-old lady has been experiencing periods of highs and lows in her mood each lasting several months at a time ever since she was a teenager. She has never previously needed psychiatric help but recently became very depressed without any obvious triggers.
2. A 29-year-old lady has been experiencing periods of elation, high energy, difficulty sleeping and excessive spending over the last 3 years. Each episode lasts about 3 weeks on average. She has had three such episodes each year on average. She has had one episodes of depression which was 3 years ago.
3. A 50-year-old man experiences chronic feelings of worrying about everything in his life – his finances, his children, his future – and he appears not to have valid reasons for such worries. He also reports that he feels depressed all the time. The depression does not appear to arise from his anxiety and he feels both the anxiety and depression are similar in extent. He says he is unsure if he feels more anxious or depressed most of the time.

1. A. Cyclothymia: ICD10 characteristics – a persistent instability of mood, involving numerous periods of mild depression and mild elation. These episodes are not sufficiently prolonged or severe to fulfil the criteria for bipolar affective disorder. This instability usually develops early in adult life and pursues a chronic course, although at times the mood may be normal and stable for months at a time.

2. D. Bipolar affective disorder: ICD10 characteristics – repeated episodes in which the patient's mood and activity levels are significantly disturbed, consisting on some occasions of elevation in mood with high energy and overactivity, and on other occasions by depression with low mood and low energy. The manic periods usually last between 2 weeks to 4–5 months. The depressive periods usually last longer (about 6 months). Rapid cycling bipolar illness is characterized by four or more episodes of hypomania, mania or depression (or a combination of these) within a 12-month period. The patient in this scenario has had three episodes per year of mania so would not fit this condition.

3. H. Mixed anxiety and depressive disorder: classified in the ICD10 under neurotic, stress-related and somatoform disorders and not under affective disorders. It is characterized by symptoms of both anxiety and depression but neither set of symptoms considered separately is severe enough to justify a diagnosis.

184. EMI – investigations in psychiatry

Options

A. Low plasma caerulo-
   plasmin
B. Hypoglycaemia
C. Hypercalcaemia
D. High urine osmolality

E. Hyperglycaemia
F. Low serum vitamin B_{12}
G. Increase in urinary
   catecholamines
H. Hyponatraemia

I. Cortical atrophy and
   hypodensities in the
   basal ganglia
J. Hypokalaemia

Instructions

For each of the scenarios described below, choose one or two of the above options that best fit. Each option may be used once, more than once or not at all.

1. A 17-year-old girl presents to the accident and emergency department with tremor and rigidity. Physical examination reveals mild jaundice and hepatomegaly (choose two).
2. A 48-year-old man has been experiencing palpitations, panic attacks, anxiety, sweating and headaches over the last 3 months without any obvious cause. Functional psychiatric illness has been ruled out (choose one).
3. A 24-year-old lady has been experiencing weight gain over the last 6 months despite her appetite being poor. She has also experienced muscle cramps as well as nausea and vomiting at times over the last few weeks. She notices her urine has become very thick orange (choose 2).

367

1. A, B. Wilson's disease: see other card for details of this condition.

2. G. Phaeochromocytoma: a very uncommon adrenal gland tumour secreting adrenaline. Symptoms include palpitations, weight loss, sweating and high blood pressure.

3. D, H: Syndrome of Inappropriate Secretion of ADH (SIADH). SIADH may be caused by: oat cell carcinoma of the lung; COAD; pancreatic cancer; Hodgkin's disease; CNS disorders – cerebral abscess, meningitis, encephalitis; myxoedema; certain drugs – antidepressants, neuroleptics, carbamazepine, diuretics, oral hypoglycaemic agents. Investigations reveal: low serum Na; elevated urine Na; low serum osmolality; high urine osmolality (highly concentrated urine).

Options

A. Lewy Body disease
B. Parkinson's disease
C. Lupus erythematosus
D. Huntington's disease

E. Hepatic encephalopathy
F. Progressive supranuclear palsy
G. Corticobasal degeneration
H. Frontotemporal dementia

Instructions

For each of the conditions described below, choose the most likely diagnosis from the list of options. Each option may be used once, more than once or not at all.

1. The patient displayed bradyphrenia, irritability and was socially withdrawn; physically he suffered from axial rigidity, and falls occurred early on during the course of the disease.
2. The 39-year-old patient was referred for psychotic symptoms, during the examination constant irregular movements of his fingers and toes were noted. He could not hold his tongue steady when asked to stick it out.
3. The 54-year-old patient was somnolent, when woken up she was not orientated to time, place or person and when asked to hold her arms and hands outstretched her hands and fingers would often briefly sink down and come up again.

1. F. Progressive supranuclear palsy (PSP): Parkinson plus syndrome, a tauopathy (abnormal formation of tau protein in the brain which may contribute to some types of dementia including frontal lobe dementia, PSP or Pick's disease) marked by axial parkinsonism, supranuclear eye movement abnormalities (vertical gaze affected), gait disorder and postural instability (falls occur early on). Cognitive disturbance, personality change and depression are also possible.

2. D. Huntington's disease: AD, trinucleotide repeat expansion (CAG), clinical picture marked by involuntary movements (chorea or other basal ganglia dysfunction), psychiatric disturbance (psychosis, depression, obsessive-compulsive symptoms, sudden outbursts of anger) and cognitive decline. 'Unsteady tongue': one possible early sign on physical examination.

3. E. Hepatic encephalopathy: manifestation variable, often seen are impairment of consciousness, confusion, visual hallucinations, mood swings (euphoria – depression); motor disorders (especially flapping tremor – asterixis as in this patient), dysarthria, ataxia, gross tremor, muscular rigidity, hyperreflexia, clonus.

Options

A. Protein 14-3-3 increased
B. Atrophy head of caudate
C. CAG expansion
D. Basilar artery distal occlusion
E. Subdural blood collection
F. Kayser–Fleischer ring
G. Raised CSF protein

Instructions

For each of the conditions described below, choose the most likely diagnosis from the list of options. Each option may be used once, more than once or not at all.

1. A 52-year-old diabetic patient developed a change of his personality during the last 24 hours and upon arrival in hospital appears excessively sleepy and is found to have a fever.
2. The patient presented with acute onset agitation and visual hallucinations while not noticing objects approaching him from the right. There is no trauma in the history.
3. A 29-year old woman has been treated for depression since her mid-twenties, she now presents with hepatosplenomegaly and thrombocytopenia. You also notice dysarthria and dystonic posturing.

1. G. Raised CSF protein: eg herpes encephalitis can present with a change in personality (71–87%). Other key symptoms are: fever (90–95%), decreased consciousness (97–100%), focal deficits (hemiparesis (33–40%), epileptic fits (62–67%)) as well as headache (74–81%) and vomiting (38–46%). CSF shows increased white cells (10–500/μl) and increased protein.

2. D. Basilar artery distal occlusion: top of the basilar artery syndrome, typical symptoms include decreased consciousness, psychosis, visual field defects, pupillary and eye movement defects, amnesia, alexia, no paresis.

3. F. Kayser–Fleischer ring: (copper deposits in the cornea) is nearly always present in patients who have developed neurological symptoms in Wilson's disease. In Wilson's disease an enzyme defect in a copper transport molecule leads to toxic levels of free copper in the serum and copper deposits in CNS, liver, kidneys and bones. The adult form of Wilson's disease presents with progressive neurological and psychiatric symptoms. Tests: ceruloplasmin (decreased), free serum copper (increased), urine 24-hour copper increased, liver biopsy, slit lamp exam.

Options

A. Akathisia
B. Tremor
C. Myoclonus
D. Ballismus

E. Chorea
F. Athetosis
G. Dystonia

H. Rigidity
I. Tics
J. Ataxia

Instructions

For each of the conditions described below, choose the presenting feature from the list of options. Each option may be used once, more than once or not at all.

1. You review a young patient with obsessive-compulsive symptoms. During the interview you notice that the patient clears his throat repeatedly and briefly straightens his shoulders on several occasions.
2. On your first contact with the patient in the outpatient department you notice sudden and irregular movement of the patient's hands and feet which seem as if the patient is playing the piano and which he also tries to incorporate into semipurposeful movements.
3. In a patient with a rapidly progressing dementing illness you observe sudden, brief, jerky movements of his left arm.

1. I. Tics: are either relatively brief, suppressable movements (motor tics) or vocalizations (vocal or phonic tics) which are preceded by a feeling of tension building up which is temporarily relieved by executing the movement/vocalization. Tics are the hallmark of Tourette's syndrome which often is associated with obsessive-compulsive symptoms, ADHD and poor impulse control.

2. E. Chorea: an involuntary, irregular hyperkinetic movement which is most prominent distally and might involve more proximal areas later in the course of the disease, eg Huntington's. Patients often try to hide the movements by incorporating them into semipurposeful gestures.

3. C. Myoclonus: an involuntary rapid stereotypical movement that can involve extremities, face and trunk. It is a feature of Creutzfeld–Jakob disease.

Options

A. Temporal lobe, dominant hemisphere
B. Temporal lobe, non-dominant hemisphere
C. Parietal lobe

D. Prefrontal cortex
E. Bilateral temporobasal

Instructions

For each of the conditions described below, where is the patient's lesion most likely located from the list of options. Each option may be used once, more than once or not at all.

1. Despite suffering from a severe left-sided hemiparesis (mainly arm and face), the patient denied any problems with his left side.
2. The patient could still discriminate between faces but he struggled to recognize them and they had lost familiarity to him.
3. The patient's behaviour was marked by hypersexuality and trying to eat nearly everything he can get hold of. He seemed easily distractible, displaying a limited range of affect and was unable to recognize objects that were shown to him.
4. The patient had lost any drive to pursue his former goals in life, often he displayed outbreaks of anger and rage and he seemed to produce a constant stream of ever-changing ideas.

1. C. Parietal lobe: neglect is most often associated with parietal lesions (R more than L) but can also occur with thalamus or basal ganglia lesions, rarely with frontal lobe lesions.

2. E. Bilateral temporobasal lobe: prosopagnosia (non-recognition of faces), here in its milder form, is usually caused by lesions either to the lower part of the visual cortex (occipital lobe) with a lesion of the underlying white matter or caused by bilateral occipitotemporobasal lesions.

3. E. Bilateral temporobasal lobe: Kluver–Bucy syndrome, bilateral temporobasal lesion, caused by: temporal lobe–tentorial herniation, herpes simplex encephalitis, transient in severe head trauma, occasionally in advanced Alzheimer's disease. Fully developed syndrome rare in humans.

4. D. Prefrontal cortex: the description given here is part of Phineas Cage's famous clinical picture after sustaining injury to the medial region of the prefrontal cortex by a tamping iron. Lesions to the prefrontal cortex can also lead to poor concentration, distractibility, loss of initiative, apathy, inability to make decisions, unpredictable and unacceptable behaviour, loss of sense of smell.

Options

A. Full blood count
B. Liver function tests
C. Paracetamol levels after 4 hours
D. Serum antimanic drug levels
E. ECG

F. Beck Depression Inventory
G. Discussion with the informant
H. Mini Mental State Exam
I. Urine drug screen

Instructions

For each of the conditions described below, state the most appropriate next step(s) from the list of options. Each option may be used once, more than once or not at all.

1. A 50-year-old man arrives at A&E after an unknown overdose. He is drowsy and gives very few answers. (3 choices)
2. A 61-year-old lady is admitted to a medical ward after a suicide attempt which she now regrets. She is taking lithium for affective disorder. (1 choice)
3. A 45-year-old man is admitted after trying unsuccessfully to hang himself. In mental state he is subjectively low in mood but objectively euthymic. He is known to misuse drugs. (3 choices)

1. B, C, E. Liver function tests, Paracetamol levels, ECG. In a drowsy patient it is important to exclude possible life-threatening overdose outcomes.

2. D. Serum antimanic drug levels

3. B, F, I. Liver function tests, Beck Depression Inventory, Urine drug screen.

Options

A. Dissociative fugue
B. Ganser's syndrome
C. Conversion disorder
D. Hypochondriasis
E. Malingering
F. Somatization disorder
G. Post-traumatic stress disorder
H. Dissociative stupor
I. Acute stress reaction
J. Adjustment disorder

Instructions

For each of the conditions described below, choose the most likely diagnosis from the list of options. Each option may be used once, more than once or not at all.

1. A 28-year-old woman presents repeatedly over the years with inexplicable chest pain. She has also complained of abdominal pain, migraine, a cough, nausea, and double vision. Various specialists have found no abnormalities.

2. A 30-year-old man complains of inexplicable pain in his abdomen. When asked questions about where he lives and his birth date his answers are slightly incorrect everytime. He has recently been made homeless. On questioning he says he can hear voices. There is inconsistency in his history.

3. A medical student approaching her finals is referred by her GP after numerous inexplicable symptoms including double vision, deafness, sensory loss and loss of pain sense. She occasionally hears 'strange noises'. She appears more concerned about her finals than the physical symptoms.

1. F. Somatization disorder: at least 2 years of multiple, recurrent, frequently changing physical symptoms with no adequate physical explanation. Persistent refusal to accept reassurance. Some impairment of social and family functioning. Usually begins before age 30. ICD10 (six symptoms relating to at least two organ systems must be present). Disorder twice as common in women.

2. B. Ganser's syndrome: rare condition, characterised by approximate answers – eg 4+4=9, psychogenic physical symptoms, hallucinations, at times clouding of consciousness, story consistently maintained. Originally described among prisoners because of obvious gain from illness. Organic illness or psychotic illness should be excluded.

3.C. Conversion disorder: term that replaced hysteria-implies conversion of problems and conflicts the individual cannot solve into symptoms. In DSM IV there are four subtypes: (1) motor symptoms or deficits; (2) sensory symptoms or deficits; (3) seizures or convulsions; (4) mixed presentation. Conversion symptoms are likely when there is no physical explanation. 'La belle indifference' (lack of concern about symptoms) has been described in conversion disorders. There may be secondary gain from symptoms – external benefits or avoidance of unwanted responsibilities.

Options

A Briquet's syndrome
B. Alcohol withdrawal
C. Delirium tremens
D. Depression
E. Fat embolism
F. Wernicke's encephalopathy
G. Tuberculosis
H. Paranoid schizophrenia
I. Schizoaffective disorder
J. Marchiafava-Bignami syndrome
K. Chronic alcohol abuse
L. Alcoholic hallucinosis

Instructions

For each of the conditions described below, choose the two most appropriate diagnoses from the list of options. Each option may be used once, more than once or not at all.

1. A 25-year-old man is suffering a bereavement. He is very anxious and finds it difficult to sleep. He is sweaty, shaking and complaining of a loss of energy, as well as suicidal thoughts.
2. A 50-year-old man is recovering on a surgical ward after a motor cycle accident. He is relatively immobile and has fractured his leg. He becomes distressed and says he is hearing voices uttering obscenities. He appears confused and disoriented and starts to experience seizures.
3. A 60-year-old man has been drinking alcohol excessively throughout most of his life. He has slurred speech, an ataxic gait, epilepsy and impaired consciousness.

1. B, D. Alcohol withdrawal and depression: Alcohol withdrawal – (i) Usually begins 12–48 hours after cessation of drinking. (ii) Common symptoms include tremor, weakness, sweating, and nausea. (iii) Seizures occur less commonly. Alcoholic hallucinosis – (i) Follows a period of abstinence after heavy chronic drinking. (ii) Characterized by auditory hallucinations usually persecutory or threatening in nature. (iii) Symptoms may last for days and can be controlled with antipsychotic drugs such as chlorpromazine.

2. C, E. Delirium tremens or fat embolism: Delirium tremens usually occurs about 7–10 days after cessation of drinking in someone in whom alcohol withdrawal has been left untreated. A serious condition which must be treated as a medical emergency. Characterized by: anxiety, confusion, difficulty sleeping; nightmares, sweating, depression; tachycardia and fever may develop; fleeting hallucinations, illusions, disorientation, visual hallucinations.

3. J, K. Marchiafava–Bignami disease (MBD) or Chronic alcohol abuse: in the more prolonged form of MBD, limb paralysis and dementia may occur. In this condition there is widespread demyelination of the optic tracts, cerebellar peduncles and corpus callosum.

Options

A. Projection
B. Displacement
C. Sublimation
D. Introjection
E. Reaction formation
F. Splitting
G. Identification with the aggressor
H. Rationalization
I. Projective identification
J. Acting out

Instructions

For each of the situations described below, choose the single most appropriate defence mechanism from the list of options. Each option may be used once, more than once or not at all.

1. A busy surgical specialist registrar has received a telling off by his consultant. Five minutes later he tells off his perplexed senior house officer over a minor matter.
2. A man is suffering acutely from a psychotic illness and has persecutory beliefs involving his mother. The mother finds herself becoming hostile and persecuting towards her son after her son shouts at her one day.
3. A man who has drug problems states that he thinks he would be able to give up his drugs more easily if his wife was more loving.

1. B. Displacement: emotions, ideas and feelings can be transferred to another person or thing, in this example to the SHO who is felt to be less important. This is a neurotic defence mechanism which can be found in phobias. Phobias represent an unconscious fear of some other situation or person.

2. I. Projective identification: a primitive defence mechanism which includes but goes beyond projection. An individual unconsciously disowns an attitude or attribute of himself and ascribes it onto another individual. Additionally, the objects of the projective identification are induced to take on and feel in a way which has been projected onto them. In the above example the mother takes on her son's aggressive thoughts and enacts them through projective identification. Although the son appears to have persecutory beliefs, it is actually his unconscious aggressive fantasies projected onto his mother.

3. H. Rationalization: this is a process of justification and reasoning after an event. An individual may provide logical explanations for his or her behaviour. The individual may try to convince others or himself of an explanation for his irrational behaviour. An external event may be blamed as a means of explanation. This along with denial is commonly seen in individuals with substance abuse.

Options

A. Paranoid schizophrenia
B. Hebephrenic schizophrenia
C. Catatonic schizophrenia
D. Simple schizophrenia
E. Undifferentiated schizophrenia

F. Schizoaffective disorder
G. Schizotypal disorder
H. Acute schizophrenia-like psychotic disorder
I. Acute polymorphic psychotic disorder
J. None of the above

Instructions

For each of the conditions described below, choose the most likely diagnosis from the list of options. Each option may be used once, more than once or not at all.

1. A young man has variations in his emotions for the first time. There has been a 10-day duration of auditory and haptic hallucinations which fluctuate from day to day.
2. A 30-year-old woman is admitted after acute ideas that the MI6 are after her. These thoughts settle quickly but her appearance and behaviour remains odd and she has overelaborate, vague speech. She has good personal functioning at home but her family have found her cold and aloof for many years.
3. A 40-year-old man has had a gradual decline in his ability to cope with life. He has taken to begging and his friends describe a once lively man who has become idle and withdrawn over the years. He does not have obvious psychotic features.

1. I. Acute polymorphic psychotic disorder: can be with or without symptoms of schizophrenia. Hallucinations and delusions vary markedly from day to day or hour to hour. Emotional turmoil, acute onset, no obvious stressors. Symptoms for less than 3 months.

2. G Schizotypal disorder: socially anxious or withdrawn, cognitive and perceptual distortions, oddities of speech and beliefs, inappropriate affect. Occasional transient quasi- psychotic episodes. Can evolve into schizophrenia, more common in individuals related to schizophrenics.

3. D Simple schizophrenia: insidious development of oddities of conduct, decline in performance and eventually may become idle and aimless. Delusions and hallucinations are less prominent. Negative symptoms develop without overt psychotic features.

Options

A. Dementia in HIV
B. Alcoholic dementia
C. Alzheimer's disease
D. Dementia in Huntington's disease
E. Pick's disease
F. Normal pressure hydrocephalus
G. Vascular dementia
H. Dementia with Lewy bodies

Instructions

For each of the conditions described below, choose the most likely diagnosis from the list of options. Each option may be used once, more than once or not at all.

1. A 65-year-old man has a history of falls and vivid images including seeing evil dwarves on waking from sleep.
2. A 75-year-old man has a history of falls. He is malnourished and unkempt. He has a mild but significant cognitive impairment.
3. A 59-year-old woman is brought in by her husband. He noticed a change in her gait, memory problems and later urinary incontinence.

1. H. Lewy body dementia: there is a fluctuating course with visual hallucinations, motor parkinsonian features, falls, syncope, delusions, auditory hallucinations and extreme sensitivity to extrapyramidal effects of antipsychotics.

2. B Alcoholic dementia: there is cognitive impairment especially when the frontal lobe is involved. CT scan shows enlarged lateral ventricles. Older patients and those drinking without respite are more at risk. Women are more at risk of cognitive impairment.

3. F. Normal pressure hydrocephalus: there is a clinical triad of early gait apraxia (broad-based gait with difficulty in initiation), bradyphrenia (slowed thinking) and later urinary incontinence. It is more common in elderly but sometimes occurs in middle life. It may be amenable to a neurosurgical shunt procedure.

Options

A. Female sex
B. Living alone
C. Having a high salary
D. Hearing impairment

E. Past history of psychiatric illness
F. High IQ
G. Recent discharge from hospital
H. Living in Greece

Instructions

For each of the conditions described below, choose three risk factors from the list of options. Each option may be used once, more than once or not at all.

1. Suicide.
2. Late-onset schizophrenia.
3. Depression.

1. B, E, G: positive associations with suicide include having a psychiatric disorder, recent discharge from hospital, chronic painful illness, previous suicide attempt or deliberate self harm, alcohol or drug abuse, male sex, being elderly, having suffered loss or bereavement, unemployment, being retired, childlessness, living alone in a city and a broken home in childhood.

2. A, B, D: late-onset schizophrenia presents after 60 with good premorbid functioning. More common in females and associated with auditory and visual deprivation. There may also be a family history of psychotic or mood disorders.

3. A, B, E: more common in females, unmarried individuals, those with a family history of depression, psychosocial stressors and physical illness.

Options

A. Autochthonous delusion
B. Secondary delusion
C. Ideas of reference
D. Thought broadcasting
E. Somatic passivity

F. Clang association
G. Tangentiality
H. Thought echo
I. Hyperacusis

J. Hyperaesthesia
K. Neologism
L. Depersonalization
M. Derealization

Instructions

For each of the conditions described below, choose two of the above options. Each option may be used once, more than once or not at all.

1. A patient on the ward is experiencing an acute relapse of her manic illness. When asked 'how are you feeling?' the patient replies 'feeling, believing, cruising like feeling and I feeling believing'. She also says she feels 'glody'.

2. An outpatient tells you he sometimes feel a sense of detachment from himself and feels like time has slowed down. While talking to you, there is a noise outside and the patient appears to find the noise very uncomfortable and distressing, saying it is very loud. The sound seems normal to the examiner.

3. A patient tells you she has pain in her abdomen and this is because your consultant has done this to her. She also says people on TV have been talking about her and she believes this because she keeps hearing her name being mentioned.

1. F, K. Clang association: rhyming and punning usually associated with acute mania with psychotic features. **Neologism:** a new word is created that has no meaning.

2. I, L. Depersonalization: a feeling of detachment from oneself, there may be an associated subjective feeling of alteration in time. **Hyperacusis:** sounds are experienced as much louder or uncomfortable than to the normal listener.

3. C, E. Somatic passivity: delusions that an external force is controlling internal bodily sensations. **Ideas of reference:** delusional belief – external cues are attributed to the self, eg hearing name on TV means people are talking about themself.

Options

A. Mitgehen
B. Mitmachen
C. Waxy flexibility
D. Negativism

E. Posturing
F. Echolalia
G. Echopraxia
H. Stupor

I. Excitement
J. Command automatism
K. Catalepsy
L. Ambitendency

Instructions

For each of the conditions described below, choose the most likely descriptions from the list of options. Each option may be used once, more than once or not at all.

1. On neurological examination, when assessing tone in the arms, the patient moves his arms excessively even if the examiner only moves the patient's arms a little.
2. Attempts at moving the patient's limbs are difficult as the patient resists movement, apparently involuntarily.
3. When the patient's arm is moved up he maintains his arm in the position in which it was placed, even though it is not in the resting position.
4. The patient carries out every instruction requested by the examiner irrespective of the consequences.

1. A. Mitgehen: excessive cooperation with passive movement.

2. D. Negativism: excessive resistance to movement.

3. C. Waxy flexibility: patient's limbs can be moved into a variety of positions and maintained thereafter for unusually long periods of time

4. J. Command automatism: instructions are performed according to instruction without concern for the consequences.

Echopraxia – automatic imitation of another person's actions.

Ambitendency – inability to complete an action without continuously starting and stopping.

Mitmachen – An individual moves their limbs or body into any position despite the examiner asking them to resist movement. When the limb(s) are released, they return to the normal position.

Stereotypy – spontaneous, repetitive, non-goal-directed movements, purposeful movements.

Options

A. Clozapine
B. Lithium
C. Quetiapine
D. Sertraline

E. Amisulpiride
F. Flupenthixol
G. Imipramine
H. Olanzapine

I. Citalopram
J. Amitriptyline
K. Paroxetine
L. Risperidone

Instructions

For each of the situations described below, choose the suitable drug(s) from the list of options. Each option may be used once, more than once or not at all.

1. Select three drugs most commonly associated with developing glucose intolerance or diabetes.
2. A young male patient complains of experiencing decreased libido and erectile dysfunction while on an antispychotic. Choose two antipsychotics that are least likely to cause sexual dysfunction.
3. A 32-year-old pregnant lady is experiencing low mood on most days as well as low energy and anhedonia. She also has low self esteem and poor sleep as well as feelings of hopelessness and worthlessness. Choose the two antidepressants above which are the safest and most used during pregnancy.
4. These antidepressants are safest for breastfeeding mothers.

1. A, B, H: about 1 in 3 patients on **clozapine** may develop diabetes after 5 years of treatment. **Lithium** may cause a reduced urinary concentrating capacity leading to nephrogenic diabetes insipidus which is reversible in the short term but may become irreversible after long term treatment (several years). **Olanzapine** is also strongly associated with a risk of diabetes.

2. C, H: quetiapine has no effect on prolactin. **Olanzapine** has minimal effects on serum prolactin.

3. G, J: imipramine and **amitriptyline** have been used although both can cause constipation and sedation. Fluoxetine has also been used but it is associated with an increased chance of early delivery and low birth weight.

4. D, K: paroxetine and **sertraline**.

199. EMI – risk factors

Options

A. Recent dose increase or reduction
B. Organic brain disease
C. Old age
D. Alcohol dependency
E. Female gender
F. Mental retardation
G. Low body weight
H. Bradycardia
I. Young age
J. Afro-Caribbean origin
K. Low white cell count
L. Hypokalaemia
M. Hyperkalaemia

Instructions

Choose the most likely risk factors from the list of options for the development of the conditions described below. Each option may be used once, more than once or not at all.

1. Neuroleptic malignant syndrome – choose four.
2. Antidepressant-induced hyponatraemia – choose three.
3. Clozapine-induced neutropenia – choose three.
4. Antipsychotic-induced QTc prolongation – choose three.

1. A, B, D, F: neuroleptic malignant syndrome is a rare side-effect which may occur with antipsychotic use. It is a potentially fatal condition if left untreated and represents a medical and psychiatric emergency. Signs and symptoms include fever, rigidity, sweating, confusion, fluctuating level of consciousness, fluctuating blood pressure and tachycardia. Blood investigations reveal raised creatine kinase (CK), leucocytosis and abnormal liver function test results. The condition must be treated urgently on the medical ward or A&E with rehydration, sedation with benzodiazepines, and bromocriptine and dantrolene may be given. ECT can be used to treat psychosis. Risk factors include: **recent rapid increase or reduction in dose**; suddenly stopping anticholinergic medication; **organic brain disease**; psychosis; **alcohol dependency**; Parkinson's disease; hyperthyroidism; **mental retardation**; psychomotor agitation.

2. C, E, G: see card 96, 'Hyponatraemia induced by antidepressants'..

3. I, J, K: 2–3% of patients treated with clozapine develop neutropenia. Risk factors include **younger age**, **Afro-Caribbean origin** and **low white cell count**.

4. H, L, M: risk factors for QTc prolongation include female gender, long QT syndrome, history of ischaemic heart disease or vascular event (eg myocardial infarction), low potassium/calcium/magnesium and physical stress.

American Psychiatric Association (1987) Diagnostic and Statistical Manual of Mental Disorders, 3rd edition, revised. Washington DC: American Psychiatric Association.

National Institute for Clinical Excellence: Clinical Guidelines. London: NICE.

Sadock BJ, Sadock VA (2003) Kaplan & Sadock's Synopsis of Psychiatry: Behavioural Sciences/Clinical Psychiatry, 9th edition. Philadelphia: Lippincott/Williams & Wilkins.

Semple D, Smyth R, Burns J, Darjee R, McIntosh A (2005) Oxford Handbook of Psychiatry. Oxford: Oxford University Press.

Taylor D, Paton C, Kerwin R (2005–2006) The Maudsley Prescribing Guidelines, 8th edition. London: The South London and Maudsley NHS Trust/Oxleas NHS Trust/Taylor and Francis Group.

World Health Organization (1992) The ICD-10 Classification of Mental and Behavioural Disorders: clinical descriptions and diagnostic guidelines. Geneva: World Health Organization.

Wright P, Stern J, Phelan M (2004) Core Psychiatry, 2nd edition. Amsterdam: Elsevier.

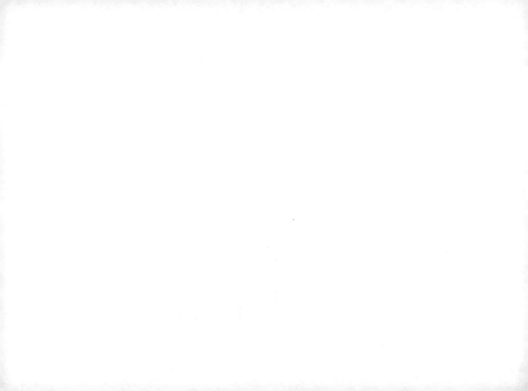

For Product Safety Concerns and Information please contact
our EU representative GPSR@taylorandfrancis.com Taylor & Francis
Verlag GmbH, Kaufingerstraße 24, 80331 München, Germany

T - #0178 - 160425 - C402 - 104/149/17 [19] - CB - 9781853156021 - Gloss Lamination